Dedicated to,
in loving memory:
For Josephine,
and Richard

Introduction

How do you integrate all the innovations that are coming your way in healthcare? How do you stay on track? How do we move towards further professionalization of the nursing profession?

In short, this book is about how nursing students can shape their vision of care from different perspectives. It gives a specific start to person-centered care, which is strongly based on building a relationship with the patient. In *Improving Person-Centered Innovation of Nursing Care: Leadership for Change*, old perspectives are erased and replaced with current, newer insights that are then brought together with passion for the nursing profession. This includes nursing care at micro, meso, and macro levels, each supported by scientific literature.

This book connects innovations in healthcare by reflecting recent insights on health and care, and connecting them from the perspective of patient-centered care. The core idea is that nurses provide care with attention to the patient as a whole. This "patient-friendly care" takes into account each patient's perceptions, preferences, and expectations when providing integrated care. Patients' experiences and needs should guide integrated care.

Care starts from the patient's point of view, as opposed to starting from the role and function of the healthcare professional. It is care where the patient is seen as a unique individual. Patients want to participate in care and do not want decisions about their health and well-being to be made without their involvement. This aspect of shared decision-making and empowerment is integrated in the book with key concepts such as relational care, holism, patient- or rather person-centered care, integrated care, quality of care, and value-based healthcare. Strategies for care and treatment should put the patient's person at the center of care and treatment.

There are no simple approaches to improve patients' quality of life, nor are there simple approaches to improve quality of (nursing) care. But an approach to quality of life and quality of care based on person-centered care can contribute to optimal (public) health.

Our current healthcare system is predominantly disease-oriented care. The emphasis is mainly on acute care (treatment of diseases, conditions, and health problems), followed by disease management with attention to risk factors (treatment of diseases and conditions). Attention to preventive care is very limited.

If we want to keep people in good health for as long as possible, the focus should be on health instead of "waiting" for (chronic) health problems to develop. Lack of time is the barrier for health professionals to shift to a health-focused approach. This requires a shift to shared knowledge. A health-focused approach requires a different orientation and approach from nursing professionals.

Improving Person-Centered Innovation of Nursing Care: Leadership for Change is written as a starting point for improving nursing care. It is written for nursing professions in both undergraduate (bachelor) and graduate (master) programs. It describes the ambition of nursing professionals to better provide every patient with the unique position in care they deserve. The book offers tools to connect important topics in education, care, and healthcare, so as to create coherence between them. Only in this way, from the perspective of person-centered care, will the professional practice of nurses be given direction.

While these topics are usually taught separately in education, this book offers the opportunity to constantly seek and recognize the interrelationship between them. This intertwining of topics is shown in Box 1, which demonstrates how we can move from an orientation on illness to person-centered care and improving health.

Love to my hommies.

Summer 2023

Box 1 Improving Person-Centered Innovation of Nursing Care: Leadership for Change

From an Orientation on Illness to Person-Centered Care with an Emphasis on improving Health.

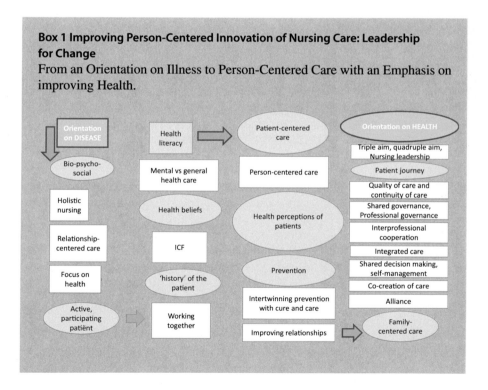

Barbara Sassen

Contents

Nursing and Holistic Care

1

1.1 Topic List for "Holistic Care: A Comprehensive Approach to Healthcare"

1. Holistic care: the interconnectedness of physical, psychological, and social aspects of health.
2. Importance of holistic nursing care: recognizing the whole person and meeting their unique needs.
3. Negative consequences of focusing solely on the biomedical aspects of health: Impaired recovery and negative health outcomes.
4. Biopsychosocial approach to care: Personalized treatment and therapy for individual needs.
5. Role of leadership in promoting holistic care: crucial for delivering high-quality care.
6. Reflecting on nursing practice: continuous evaluation of nursing actions for effective care.
7. Shortcomings of a disease-specific medical model: overlooking the patient as a whole person.
8. Patient-centered care: shifting from a disease-focused to a person-centered approach.
9. Importance of therapeutic relationship: caring approach with respect and positivity towards patients.
10. Multimorbidity and complex care needs: challenges in disease-specific healthcare system, insufficient care for this patient population, higher risk of negative health effects, and decreased quality of life.
11. Increased healthcare utilization and costs for patients with multimorbidity.
12. Importance of addressing multimorbidity in holistic care: comprehensive approach for better patient outcomes and satisfaction.

B. Sassen, *Improving Person-Centered Innovation of Nursing Care*, https://doi.org/10.1007/978-3-031-35048-1_1

1.2   Introduction

Holistic care is an approach that considers the whole person, including their physical, psychological, and social aspects, as interrelated and interdependent. By adopting a holistic approach, healthcare professionals can better understand how illness affects patients and respond to their real needs. On the other hand, a narrow focus on biological health without considering the psychological and social impacts of illness can hinder recovery and lead to adverse health outcomes. This chapter explores the importance of holistic care in nursing. Culture plays a vital role in healthcare, and healthcare professionals must take cultural diversity into account when providing care to their patients. Culturally competent care is an approach that ensures healthcare providers are aware of the cultural values and norms of their patients, and their families, and provides care accordingly. Primary nursing has emerged as a critical aspect of patient care, emphasizing the importance of the nurse–patient relationship and personalized care for each patient. In this context, patient-centered care can be used as a strategy to tailor care to the patient's unique needs and improve health outcomes.

1.3   Outline

This chapter is about the concept of holistic care in nursing. It explains that holistic care considers the whole person and assumes that the biopsychosocial aspects mutually influence one another. It is important to start from a holistic view of humanity and approach the patient or client as a holistic unit. The biomedical component focuses on medical care and eliminating the illness, while the psychological component considers the patient as a unique individual with their own needs, wishes, and expectations. The social component involves looking at the patient in their social-emotional context. The chapter also discusses the impact of multimorbidity on healthcare and how healthcare professionals should follow multiple guidelines for multimorbidity because care is often insufficiently geared towards patients with multimorbidity. Finally, it highlights the importance of person-centered care and a caring therapeutic relationship between healthcare professionals and patients.

1.4   Holistic Care

Holistic care involves a comprehensive approach to healthcare that considers the interconnectedness of a person's physical, psychological, and social aspects. This approach enables nurses to gain a better understanding of how illness affects the whole person and how to meet their specific needs (Mead and Bower 2000). Focusing solely on the biological aspects of health, without considering the psychological and social impact of illness, can impede recovery and lead to negative health outcomes (Suhonen et al. 2000, as cited in Morgan and Yoder 2012).

Therefore, it is an essential part of nursing care to approach patients as holistic individuals, recognizing their unique complexities. By adopting a biopsychosocial approach to care, everyone can receive personalized treatment and therapy that addresses their specific needs. It is important to view every patient as a holistic unit to provide meaningful care that promotes recovery and improves overall well-being.

As a nurse, leadership is crucial in promoting holistic care and treatment. Additionally, providing excellent patient care necessitates reflecting on one's own nursing practice. Continuously evaluating the effectiveness and necessity of nursing actions is critical to delivering high-quality care

Unfortunately, many people, both inside and outside the healthcare sector, tend to approach patient care from a purely medical perspective, focusing solely on available treatment options. This approach overlooks the fundamental truth that a human being is more than their health problems. Although every individual seeking healthcare has specific needs due to their illness, they also expect to be recognized and treated as a whole person, not just as a collection of symptoms.

Task-oriented nursing care has long been a standard practice in the nursing profession, aligning with a medical perspective on health and care. However, when an individual becomes ill, it affects their entire being. Even limiting the consequences of illness can greatly benefit patients. Illness impacts all aspects of a person's life, including their ability to work or study, to fulfill personal aspirations, to maintain relationships, and to enjoy life. It can cause physical and emotional suffering, leading to despair and anxiety.

To adopt a holistic view of patient care and treatment, it is crucial to consider the patient as a biopsychosocial entity. This means understanding the interplay between the biomedical, psychological, and social aspects of their health and well-being, as illustrated in Fig. 1.1. Each of these components must be considered and addressed to provide comprehensive care.

Seen from a biomedical model, it concerns medical care. If you start from a medical point of view and look at the patient's illness, the attention is focused on eliminating that illness. The disease is the starting point. Care and treatment the solution to handle the disease.

In the past, patients were often expected to play a passive role in their healthcare. When healthcare providers asked "Any questions?" at the end of a consultation, patients frequently responded with a simple "No." However, the traditional, disease-specific medical model, which was centered around the healthcare provider, has shifted to a more personalized approach that is tailored to each individual patient (Morgan and Yoder 2012). In the past, the healthcare system was organized around medical professionals, rather than around the patient. The origins of this patient-centered concept may be traced back to Florence Nightingale, who distinguished nursing from medicine by emphasizing the importance of focusing on the patient rather than just the disease.

Carl Rogers built upon this concept with his emphasis on person-centered care (Morgan and Yoder 2012). Rogers believed that every person has the capacity to

Fig. 1.1 Client-centered
holistic approach

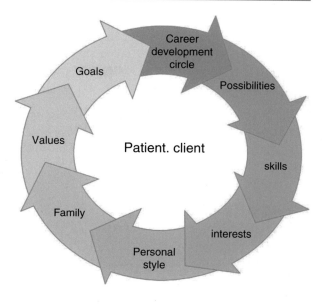

Fig. 1.2 Biopsychosocial
health . (beeldrechten:
[rechten bij auteur],
bestand:)

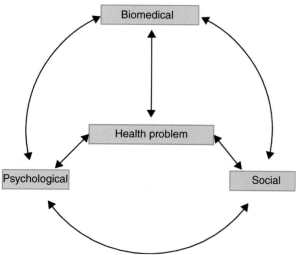

heal, provided that they receive appropriate support and are approached with respect and positivity. This involves healthcare professionals entering into a caring therapeutic relationship with their patients, rather than viewing them as objects of disease. Patients should be recognized as individuals with unique social and emotional contexts, as illustrated in Fig. 1.2 (Mead and Bower 2000).

Multimorbidity refers to the co-occurrence of multiple health problems in a patient, often resulting in complex care needs. However, our healthcare system is predominantly disease-specific and tends to focus on addressing individual health problems, as depicted in Fig. 1.3. As a result, when patients present with multiple

Fig. 1.3 Disease-specific orientation. (beeldrechten: [rechten bij auteur], bestand:)

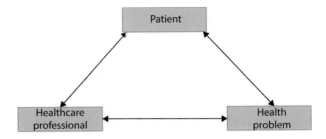

health problems or complex care needs, our healthcare system may be less equipped to provide the appropriate care.

Healthcare professionals often work in a disease-specific manner, following guidelines that are specific to each individual health condition. However, these guidelines do not typically provide guidance for managing patients with multimorbidity, who often require more complex care. As a result, there may be a lack of adequate care for this patient population. Despite the significant impact that having multiple chronic illnesses can have on a patient's well-being, the current healthcare system is insufficiently geared towards providing care for patients with multimorbidity. This can result in unfavorable patient outcomes, including a higher risk of negative health effects and even death. Additionally, patients with multimorbidity tend to use healthcare facilities more frequently, resulting in higher costs. Furthermore, research has shown that patients with multimorbidity often report a lower quality of life and are less satisfied with their care (Kuipers et al. 2019).

From a psychological perspective, taking a holistic view of a patient involves recognizing their unique individuality. Each patient has their own distinct needs, wishes, and expectations. Illness can significantly impact a patient's self-perception and how they view themselves. For example, if a person previously saw themselves as healthy, experiencing an illness can result in a shift towards identifying as someone who is sick. This may require the patient to re-evaluate their entire sense of self. However, more commonly, a patient's view changes to acknowledging that their health is faltering, but they are still the same person they were before.

Illness and health are deeply personal concepts that are viewed differently by each individual. From a biopsychosocial perspective, the psychological aspects of a patient's experience are an integral component. From a sociological perspective, individuals are part of social groups that significantly influence their lives. The patient's social environment, and the groups to which they belong, can impact their experience of illness. When a patient's health is faltering, their ability to participate in social roles may be affected. Patients often have roles to fulfill within their family, workplace, and community, such as being a spouse, parent, grandparent, child, or student. Illness can impact their ability to fulfill these roles and participate in social activities.

The sociological perspective is focused on the social functioning of individuals, including how they function within their social environment when they are ill. The values and norms that are present within these social groups can influence how a patient views their own health and illness. When considering the patient as a biopsychosocial unit, the sociological perspective covers these social aspects of health and illness.

In addition to the biopsychosocial model, the spiritual perspective can also be considered. Holistic care should be tailored to the individual patient, considering their religious beliefs and coping mechanisms, as well as their spiritual well-being and needs. Many patients place great importance on their spiritual needs, particularly during the final phase of life (Sulmasy 2002). Holistic care prioritizes human dignity, and can help to improve the patient's self-awareness and self-confidence. Palliative care is an important aspect of holistic care that can enhance the patient's quality of life.

Holistic care involves planning and providing care based on all four perspectives, as discussed above (refer to Fig. 1.4). This includes taking into consideration individual patient needs and stressors in their life (Lor et al. 2016). Holistic care also emphasizes interprofessional and coordinated care, with the aim of achieving optimal quality of life for the patient (Ventegodt et al. 2016).

Providing care solely based on the medical model often leads to longer hospital stays and higher healthcare costs (Zamanzadeh et al. 2015). The medical model relies on routines and may not sufficiently address the patient's individual needs. It is crucial that healthcare professionals possess empathy and a deep understanding of their patients, as this can lead to a more holistic approach to care (McEvoy and Duffy 2008).

The patient's social environment, including family and community, plays a crucial role in their well-being and ability to cope with illness. For nurses to provide effective, patient-centered care, it is essential to involve the patient's important

Fig. 1.4 Holistic care.
(beeldrechten: [rechten bij
auteur], bestand:)

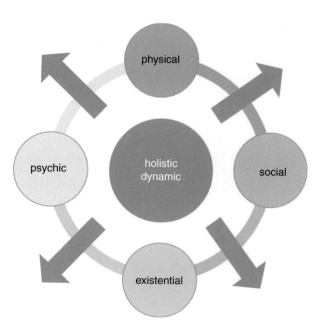

relationships. In the case of chronic health problems, the social environment can significantly influence how the patient copes with their illness and integrates it into their life.

Social support can be informal or formal, with peer support from significant others having a significant impact on health outcomes and behaviors. Peer support can positively affect the treatment of chronic health problems and reduce the time healthcare professionals need to spend with patients (WHO 2003).

Families often provide informal care and play a vital role in the psychosocial context, especially for patients with chronic health problems and elderly care. In palliative care, the patient and their family form a dynamic unit, and healthcare professionals should be sensitive to family connections (Fleming et al. 2006).

Families play a dual role in caring for patients—as caregivers and care partners. They provide support in daily activities, accompany patients to appointments, and can even play a role in the care treatment process. For instance, care partners of people with Parkinson's disease report symptoms more frequently than the patients themselves (Rastgardani et al. 2019). Without the help of family, patients could not receive complete treatment. Moreover, families have a unique view of the symptoms and effects of treatment, recognizing emotional, physical, and psychosocial needs.

The family's role should be integrated into patient-centered care, as they can monitor health status, clarify and prioritize care goals when patients cannot speak for themselves. In such cases, the family should also be involved in the preparation of the care plan and should have the opportunity to consult with the professional team. A systematic review found that families would like to be involved in decision-making but often feel left out by professionals (Yamanishi et al. 2013).

Although family and friends can help patients during their illness, nursing professionals often face barriers to involving them in care and providing support. They are concerned about properly safeguarding patient privacy and experience it as an extra task burden. Healthcare professionals also often feel insecure about their capacity to interact with family and friends. Rastgardani et al. (2019) argue that healthcare professionals should provide support to family and friends in their role as care partners.

The values and standards that are culturally determined by a patient can significantly impact the quality of care they receive. When healthcare providers take into account the patient's cultural background and that of their family, it is known as culturally competent care. By understanding culture-specific norms, values, and factors that contribute to cultural beliefs, healthcare professionals gain insight into providing culturally competent care, which may also require exploring health literacy. Culturally competent care enhances patient trust and encourages their active participation in their care, leading to better health outcomes and patient self-management. Additionally, it decreases stress and improves the patient's mental health, as well as increases satisfaction for both the patient and their family and fosters a better relationship between the healthcare professional and the patient (Lor et al. 2016).

Cultural diversity refers to the social differences between various cultural groups, which can sometimes pose challenges in communication and building cooperative relationships. Cultural patterns are the social customs, values, and behaviors that are transmitted from one generation to the next and play a vital role in shaping people's identities.

To provide more patient-centered care, primary nursing has emerged as an alternative to task-oriented care. The nurse–patient relationship is critical for ensuring the continuity and quality of care. With primary nursing, a single nurse collaborates with the patient to oversee the entire nursing process. This process starts with the nurse's review of the patient's medical history, followed by the formulation of broad, clustered nursing and interprofessional diagnoses. The nursing care plan is then customized to the patient's unique situation and biopsychosocial needs. Finally, the nursing care is organized, with regular feedback loops to the medical history to adjust care as the patient's needs change due to health or psychosocial reasons. The planning and implementation of (interprofessional) nursing interventions are personalized to meet the patient's needs and are based on a health problem and pattern approach that can be carried out by any nursing professional.

The final step of the nursing process involves evaluating the care provided to the patient. This evaluation involves assessing the care treatment process and determining with the patient whether adjustments need to be made to the care and patient management. A visual analogue scale (VAS) can be utilized in this evaluation, on which patients can indicate their perceived quality of life, extent of person-centered care, level of comfort, and pain experience. Evaluation is also conducted at the time of discharge or referral, during which the care plan is reviewed, and the care and treatment provided are discussed with the patient. The goal of this final evaluation is to obtain feedback for quality improvement.

The primary process, from admission to discharge, involves the provision of care by nurses or other professionals in a multidisciplinary team (Dwamena et al. 2012; Hirsch et al. 2013; Rostgardani 2019). Patient-centered care can be used as a strategy to tailor care to the patient throughout the entire nursing process and influence treatment choices. It is important to prioritize the patient's needs and preferences and involve them in decision-making for optimal care outcomes (Dwamena et al. 2012).

1.5 Conclusion

- In conclusion, holistic care is an essential aspect of nursing that recognizes the complexity of human beings and acknowledges the interrelatedness of their physical, psychological, and social aspects. The biomedical, psychological, and social components of the holistic approach highlight the importance of seeing the patient as an individual in their social-emotional context and addressing their unique needs, wishes, and expectations.
- By adopting a holistic view of humanity and approaching patients as biopsychosocial units, healthcare professionals, especially nurses, can provide high-quality care that leads to better health outcomes and higher patient satisfaction.

- Continuous reflection on nursing practices and leadership in shaping holism in professional care is crucial to ensure that patients receive the best care possible.
- Providing culturally competent care and adopting a patient-centered approach can improve patient confidence, willingness to participate in care, and ultimately, their health outcomes.
- Primary nursing emphasizes the importance of the nurse–patient relationship and personalized care for each patient, while evaluation at each step of the nursing process allows for continuous improvement and ensures the provision of quality care. Overall, healthcare providers must provide care that meets their specific needs to ensure the best possible patient outcomes.

Box 1.1 Mind-Map Holistic View of Humanity
Create a mind-map on the importance of a holistic approach to nursing care. Point out why it is crucial for nursing professionals to approach patients as a holistic unit, and: how this approach can improve the quality of care provided. The sub-aspects of the biomedical, psychological, and social components of a holistic view of humanity could be explored.

Box 1.2 Mind-Map Leadership in Shaping Holistic Nursing Care
Create a mind-map on the role of leadership in shaping holism in nursing care. Point out: which (leadership) skills nurses need to develop, to promote a holistic approach to nursing care?

Box 1.3 Mind-Map on Challenges in Providing Holistic Care for Patients with Multimorbidity
Create a mind-map on challenges in providing care for patients with multimorbidity. Point out: explore the challenges healthcare professionals face in providing holistic care to patients with multiple health problems at the same time.

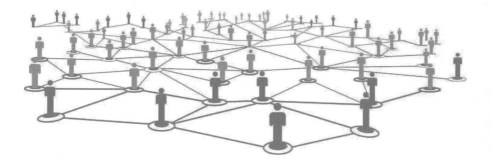

Nursing and Relationship-Based Nursing

2

2.1   Topic List

1. The challenges of developing a collaborative relationship and establishing a bond with patients due to limited time during contact moments.
2. The importance of providing holistic care that addresses the biopsychosocial needs of patients.
3. The impact of neglecting psychosocial aspects of illness and patient management on care quality.
4. The link between effective cooperation during contact moments and improved adherence to treatment.
5. The changing power dynamics between healthcare professionals and patients, with patients being seen as the center of care.
6. The shift from a professional-centered focus to a patient-centered approach in healthcare.
7. The role of the internet in changing the access to medical knowledge and empowering patients to be more involved in their own health.
8. The need for a shift in thinking about health and illness, with a focus on expanding health and investing in prevention and health promotion.
9. The importance of recognizing patients as unique individuals beyond their diseases.
10. The concept of relational, person-centered care as a way of providing high-quality care in healthcare settings.
11. The principles of nursing, including the foundation of building relationships with patients and clients.
12. The challenges and barriers to implementing relational, person-centered care in healthcare practice.

B. Sassen, *Improving Person-Centered Innovation of Nursing Care*,
https://doi.org/10.1007/978-3-031-35048-1_2

2.2   Introduction

Providing high-quality healthcare services requires a holistic approach, where the patient is viewed as a biopsychosocial unit. However, healthcare professionals tend to focus only on the physical and biological aspects of illness, forgetting to include the psychosocial aspects in care and treatment. Collaboration and establishing a bond with the patient are crucial for the successful management of health problems. In this regard, the time factor in contact moments can be a hindrance but emphasizing collaboration on practical aspects of care and treatment may offer a way to compensate for this.

2.3   Outline

The chapter discusses the importance of a patient-centered approach in healthcare. It highlights that while professionals recognize the importance of providing holistic care and patient-centered care. The power relationship between medical professionals and patients has changed due to the internet, and patients are now more assertive and informed. The text argues that the focus should be on the patient as the center of care, with an approach of equality and collaboration, respecting the rights and autonomy of the patient. The text suggests that expanding health and recognizing health risks and anticipating them with prevention and health promotion can significantly benefit patients. The concept of relational, person-centered care provision is discussed, which involves entering into a relationship with the patient and tailoring care to their unique needs. The text emphasizes the need for an attitude of empathy and responsiveness towards the patient and their family in healthcare.

2.4   Relationship-based Nursing

Although the limited time available during contact moments can pose a challenge to developing a collaborative relationship and establishing a bond with the patient, focusing on practical aspects of care and treatment can help compensate for this (Thompson and McCabe 2012). Healthcare professionals recognize the importance of providing holistic care that addresses the patient's biopsychosocial needs and aim to deliver patient-centered care. However, they often neglect the psychosocial aspects of illness and patient management, leading to suboptimal care (McCormack et al. 2010; Ekman et al. 2011). Effective cooperation during contact moments in both general and mental health care has been linked to improved adherence, and positive relationships or alliances with patients have been shown to enhance therapy adherence (Thompson and McCabe 2012).

The biopsychosocial model teaches nurses to approach every patient with a holistic perspective. The starting point of good care provision is that the nurse makes contact with the patient and enters into a relationship with him (Fig. 2.1). For high-quality care, it is about relational care (Baart 2018). Nurses look at care from

Fig. 2.1 Shared
partnership (Arnold and
Underman Boggs 2020).
(beeldrechten: [rechten bij
auteur], bestand:)

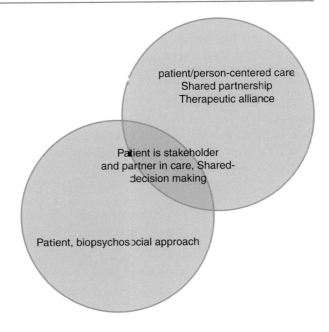

patient/person-centered care
Shared partnership
Therapeutic alliance

Patient is stakeholder
and partner in care, Shared-
decision making

Patient, biopsychosocial approach

their knowledge of the general needs of people. Then they look at the specific patient
and what their needs are. Relational caregiving involves both a general level and a
specific level and together this forms unique caregiving. Nurses should work on
doing the right thing and tailoring the right thing to the person (Baart 2018).

The consequence of the development that patients have access to more and more
medical information and are also more assertive than in the past is that the power
relationship between the medical professional and the patient has changed. The
focus should be shifted, whereby the patient is now seen as the center of care. This
means a turnaround in thinking about health and illness. All of us, as a society,
should invest more in health: not just because of the financial benefits, but above all
from a vision and professional perspective. The adage "you are healthy until you are
sick" no longer applies, but "stay healthy even when you are sick."

In healthcare, a professional-centered focus has long existed. The focus was
"you are healthy until you are sick." Moving this focus to the patient as the center
of care is imperative. Although healthcare professionals said that the well-being of
the patient is paramount, there was an imbalance of power in which professionals
assumed they knew what was best for the patient and the patient had to act
accordingly. This paternalistic attitude has been replaced by an approach of equality
and collaboration, respecting the rights and autonomy of the patient (Gill et al. 2019).

The balance of power between the medical profession and the patient has
changed. Medical progress has led to accurate diagnoses and effective and efficient
treatments. This created the impression that medical health problems could be
solved with science and technology and that the knowledge in this area lay with the
medical profession. But this position is shifting due to the internet, which not only

makes medical knowledge available to everyone, but also allows more and more people to use, interpret and apply it to deal with illness and health.

There should be a shift in thinking about health and illness. We should invest more in health. Not only financially, but especially from a vision and professional perspective.

This is about expanding health. Many health problems cannot simply be brushed away with medicines and some healthcare; many health problems are or become chronic. People are getting older and older, so it is to be expected that being sick, having one or more chronic health problems, is or will become part of life. It is precisely in this area that significant health benefits can be achieved by investing in health. By expanding health, you can expect health benefits and well-being. Attention should be focused much more on keeping every patient happy and healthy. This by focusing on expanding health and the early recognition of health risks, by improving prevention and health promotion (Sassen 2018a).

> … shared partnership in which the patient is an equal stakeholder and treatment partner in ensuring quality health care … (Arnold and Underman Boggs 2020).

We have abandoned the idea that the patient is his disease. The patient is more than their disease. If you ask the patients themselves, they will mainly say that they are people with a disease. Although this disease determines their lives to a greater or lesser extent, it does not stop them from leading their own lives. In the health care sector, patients used to be referred to by names such as diabetes patients, depressed patients, kidney patients, rheumatic patients, and schizophrenic patients. Now we say about people with diabetes, people with depressive symptoms, people with ... Nursing care is primarily about this person as a person, then the attention is focused on how we can offer this person the right care as a unique person.

Relational, person-centered care provision is a way of providing good care and is in fact the counterpart of task-oriented care provision. Whereas in the past the emphasis was on task-oriented care provision, with the focus on providing care on sub-aspects of care and certain tasks with the patient, this has shifted to primary nursing.

For primary nursing, entering a relationship is the foundation on which care is built. This can be care by an individual nurse, but more often it will be a small team of nursing professionals who take care of the entire care process. This form of care is characterized by an attitude of empathy and responsiveness of the care professionals, towards the patient and his family.

Although the concept of primary, relational nursing seems obvious, this principle is not applied straight forward. It turns out to differ between nursing professionals and occurs in a random, non-systematic way (Korhonen and Kangasniemi 2013). Consistent planning, implementation, and evaluation also appear not to be integrated as standard and systematically (Naef et al. 2019). Providing person-centered care is not easy. It is easy to smile and say hi, but it gets more complicated when decisions must be made, responding appropriately and matching the patient's preferences, values, and needs, and responding appropriately every time (Gill et al. 2019).

In the model of primary nursing, it is essentially about the trinity of person-centered care, coordinated care, and continuous care. The primary nursing model revolves around person-centered, patient-based professional nursing care, in which the primary nurse takes responsibility for the coordination and continuity of patient-centered care processes and patient-centered professional care (Naef et al. 2019).

Primary, relationship-oriented nursing has a strong orientation on patient- or person-oriented nursing. Person-centered care ensures that continuity in contact with the nurse is experienced. This involves shared decision-making as well as coordinated care where healthcare professionals work together in multidisciplinary teams throughout the patient's admission.

For patient-centered care in the primary nursing model, the autonomy of the nurse and the display of leadership as a professional regarding the care to be provided is fundamental. In addition, for patient-centered care in the model of primary nursing, clinical reasoning and clinical decision-making are the foundations for the desired nursing care (Wessel et al. 2017).

If nurses propagate their autonomous function from leadership and let clinical reasoning be the point of departure for their nursing care, primary nursing can lead to "care satisfaction," greater satisfaction with care and to more job satisfaction for nursing professionals themselves.

Going forward, due to the increase in complex care needs of patients, primary care will be the foundation of teams working together to provide integrated and coordinated care, both within and across healthcare settings.

In a focus group study, key elements related to patient-centered care were identified. This concerns the importance of building a relationship with the patient, providing individualized care to the patient and respecting the patient's time (Gray et al. 2019).

The first is the importance of building a relationship with the patient. Building a relationship means that you, as a nursing professional, enter into a partnership with the patient. You look for opportunities to work together with the patient and his family and ask for their input. Key points for building a relationship with the patient include:

- spending sufficient time;
- listening with attention;
- showing an emphatic attitude;
- making verbal and non-verbal contact;
- communicating in an honest and transparent way;
- responding without judging the patient;
- respecting the privacy of the patient.

Secondly, it is about providing individualized care to the patient. For personalized care, elements are that such care can be provided by knowing the patient. For this it is also important to involve the family. In personalized care, the nurse should be understanding the patient's personal circumstances. To this end, it may be important to clarify the patient's words, as well as to respond culturally competent and sensitively.

Third, the importance of respecting patient time. Respecting the time of the patient and his family involves waiting times, ensuring that patients can make appointments easily, ensuring that patients are called back in a timely manner, and so on.

Patients who are actively involved in care and treatment, and in decision-making, manage their health and disease better. This means that they deal better with it, that they manage their health problem better in line with guidelines and protocols.

In line with the patient as an active partner in healthcare, new initiatives are needed in areas such as eHealth and patient records, so that patients can not only view their patient data, but also add data if desired.

2.5   Conclusion

- The balance of power between the medical profession and the patient or client has shifted, and it is imperative to move the focus from the healthcare professional to the patient or client as the center of care. Healthcare professionals should respect the rights and autonomy of the patient and adopt an approach of equality and collaboration.
- By focusing on relational, person-centered care provision, healthcare professionals can offer the right care to each patient as a unique person.
- Investing in health and expanding health can result in significant health benefits and well-being.
- Ultimately, a shared partnership in which the patient is an equal stakeholder and treatment partner in ensuring quality health care can lead to positive outcomes in healthcare management.

Box 2.1 Mind-Map Importance of Collaboration in Patient Care
Create a mind-map on the importance of collaboration in patient care. Point out: how can you as a nursing professional develop a positive relationship or alliance with the patient. And, how one can work on doing the right thing?

Box 2.2 Mind-Map Shift in Power Relationship
Create a mind-map on the shift in power relationship between the medical professional and the patient: the medical profession has long existed in a professional-centered focus, where the patient was seen as healthy until sick. Point out: How to shift the focus to the patient being the center of care?

Nursing and the Patient's Illness Experience

3

3.1 Topic List: When People Become Ill, the Perspective on Life Changes

1. The veil of gray: how Illness Can Diminish the Luster of Life.
2. Uncertainty and Recovery: navigating the Unknowns of Chronic Illness.
3. Building a Relationship with the Patient: dignity and Respect in Nursing Practice.
4. Alienation and Disconnect: addressing patients' feelings of separation in healthcare.
5. The changing landscape of doing the Right Thing: contextual care in healthcare.

3.2 Introduction

The experience of illness can have a profound effect on a person's perspective on life, with a veil of gray descending on what was once a sunny existence. While some illnesses may be temporary, others can become chronic, casting a permanent shadow on the patient's life. Disease can cause a twilight state, leaving patients or clients uncertain about the future and struggling with fear, anxiety, and disbelief. Healthcare professionals have an important role to play in supporting patients through this difficult time, providing respectful and patient-specific care that acknowledges the patient's dignity and empowers them to make informed decisions about their health.

3.3 Outline

The content of this chapter discusses the impact of illness on a person's life, both in terms of physical and emotional effects. It explains that illness can cause a veil of gray over one's life, and chronic illness can permanently affect the patient's experience of life. The passage also emphasizes the importance of healthcare

B. Sassen, *Improving Person-Centered Innovation of Nursing Care*, https://doi.org/10.1007/978-3-031-35048-1_3

professionals doing the right thing by providing patient-centered care that is tailored to the patient's needs and context. This includes building a respectful relationship with the patient, offering choices, and providing person-specific support. Relational caregiving is emphasized to address the feelings of alienation that illness can evoke. Finally, this chapter discusses the potential for patients to feel disconnected from their healthcare due to the fragmented nature of the healthcare system and emphasizes the importance of building relationships with patients to counteract this.

3.4   Illness Experience

When people become ill, the perspective on life will change. People can experience that "a big storm" has started in their lives. Or at least that life is less sunny than they experienced before. To a greater or lesser extent, people will experience a veil of gray over their lives and experience that the shine of their lives has been lost. An illness can be temporary, after which the veil of gray disappears, and the splendor of life can return. However, illness can also become chronic, so that the gray veil and reduced luster always, to a greater or lesser extent, have an influence on the patient.

Disease can evoke a kind of twilight state in the patient. For a short or longer period of time they may not fully realize what exactly is happening in their lives. This can cause stress, they can experience fear and anxiety, or disbelief.

Patients and clients are in uncertainty: will my disease ever pass? Even if the problem appears to have been averted and recovery has occurred, the patient carries the event with him. This has an influence on his life and continues to have this influence on a greater or lesser extent. The veil of gray has become diffuse, but the shine often does not return completely. "I am better again" will often not mean that the patient feels and lives again as he did before the health complaints. Life has changed because of the illness experience. The patient will have to learn to live with what it is like to be a person with a health problem.

Healthcare professionals should do the right thing. Doing the right thing means doing what is right in the context in which care is provided. Doing the right thing then means: doing what is good for this person, in this situation and at this moment (Baart 2018). The care is then properly geared to the context (for example, the family situation), is good for this person (for example, a cancer patient in the palliative phase of illness), in this situation (for example, the home situation) and at this moment. Doing the right thing, therefore, fluctuates and changes over time. It is strongly linked to the patient–nurse relationship.

Building a relationship with the patient is reflected in the way you deal with the patient's dignity. It is about respectful nursing behavior. This means that as a healthcare professional you are prepared to listen to the patient and that you pay attention to the perspectives and choices of the patient and his family (Gray et al. 2019). The dignity of the patient and treating him with respect is the starting point for nursing practice. It is reflected in the way of making contact with the patient, inviting the patient to participate from the first moment of contact and throughout the entire care treatment process ("We would like to hear your opinion and will often ask for it…"). After all, maintaining good contact is the basis for reaching joint decision-making.

Respectful care provision means that each patient is seen as competent to make decisions regarding their own care (Leplege et al. 2007). We should see patients as active healthcare consumers who have the right to choose health services and care for themselves (Mead and Bower 2000). Providing choices is a form of respectful care that is important to every person. It stimulates patients' strength and offers the opportunity to be and remain independent (Morgan and Yoder 2012). Yoder-Wisse (2019) also mentions that consumer relationships play a central role in nursing care and health care as a whole.

Healthcare professionals should provide patient-specific, informative support to patients. This means that they should share all information related to a patient with him or her. And that this information is unbiased, no information is left out and delivered in a way that is supportive and useful for the patient and his family. This informative support must also be provided in a timely manner, because only complete and accurate information offers the possibility to participate in care and decision-making. Only when the patient and his family have all the information, i.e., about the disease process and procedures, about the health aspects, about test results, about support and follow-up, can they make informed decisions about their own health situation (Gray et al. 2019).

Relational caregiving is not about a set of consecutive actions. Relational care provision is about entering into a relationship with the patient and taking this as a starting point for good care. Illness can evoke feelings of alienation in the patient. Illness always raises questions for the patient. Why? Why is this happening to me? Some patients take this one step further and wonder: What did I do to deserve this? What did I do that this happened to me? These unsettling feelings need to be discussed with the patient. Nursing professionals should aim to recognize these reactions and discuss them with the patient. Within relational nursing, the discussion of these feelings that evoke alienation can be given a place within the care provision. More often this should be a recurring topic of conversation.

It is not only the experience of illness itself that gives the patient feelings of alienation from his own person, his body, and his entire social functioning. In this modern age of specialist care and scaling up, patients increasingly feel disconnected from their own healthcare. The contacts that the patient has with the health care system can lead to the patient experiencing feelings of alienation. The patient may feel alienated from himself and from his environment. A number of reasons can be identified for this.

Within the healthcare sector, contacts are often fleeting, with several professionals from the various disciplines involved in the care of an individual patient. While the general practitioner is often known to the patient in his care, contacts with healthcare professionals can be short term and therefore more volatile if his health problem requires further investigation and treatment in a (psychiatric) hospital. By entering into a relationship with the patient as a nurse and by providing care in a relational atmosphere, the patient can feel more connected to his own health.

Nurses should use the relationship with the patient as a means to deal with feelings of alienation. But how do you do that? What does not work is if the nurse chooses "reassurance" as a strategy to "mute" the patient's feelings. Patients are skeptical about this, especially when the treatment lasts longer and favorable results are not achieved. Patients do not need reassurance if they express their concern. What they do need is to talk about their concerns. But that is only possible if they have established a relationship with a nurse who is open to this. Only then can this nurse give the patient the feeling that he is being listened to as a person. The nurse should really be interested in how the patient experiences his illness. The patient should feel the space to discuss his concerns, he should feel heard. A patient does not expect you to solve their problems (Sassen 2018, 2023).

Nurses should work in partnership with the patient, within interprofessional care teams. The alignment between nurses and the patient is about seeing the patient as a holistic, biopsychosocial unit, in contact with his family and friends. The nurse works from the collaborative relationship with the patient by using an effective communication style, offering respectful care from a holistic perspective, individual-oriented. The nurse is focused on empowerment, and is family oriented. Within the interprofessional team, the nurse works on the interprofessional coordination of care. Interpersonal relationships are an important starting point for care, with the nurse having sufficient culturally supported knowledge and skills to provide depth to the care. It is not unimportant that the nurse conveys a sense of social justice in her professional practice (Fig. 3.1).

Developing recovery strategies in care plans could be useful here. The patient can make a well-informed choice, for example, for the transition from hospital to home situation. For recovery, it is important to develop client-centered care plans, to set goals, to focus on aspects of daily living and to identify what support the patient needs after discharge. These care plans, and especially the involvement of the patient in them, can stimulate the patient's interest in his personal well-being (Cleary et al. 2012b).

Entering a relationship with the patient, partner with patients, can take shape by offering coaching, giving support and advice, acknowledging the patient's own role and responsibility, and—time and time again—determining what needs priority (Gray et al. 2019).

Maximizing communication technology is desirable in the healthcare sector. Here, too, the needs of the patient and his family should be the starting point. This involves exploring options, providing support in the knowledge of the patient and his family, to be able to prioritize care and treatment and to make decisions (Gray et al. 2019).

A review shows that partnership, together with good communication and health promotion, are the core elements of patient-centered care (Constand et al. 2014). In a patient-centered approach, professionals can choose which of these three core elements best fits or should take precedence in the given situation with a particular patient. For patient-centered care, good communication is the most important, next to partnership and health promotion (Constand et al. 2014).

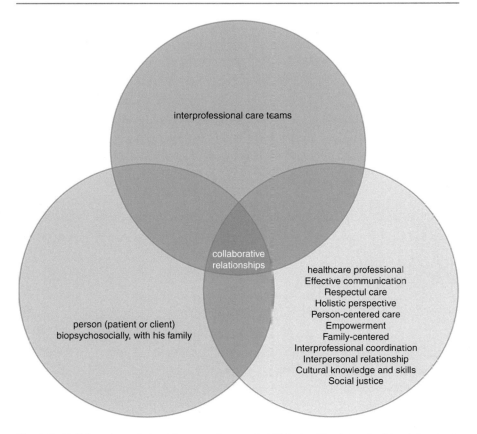

interprofessional care teams

collaborative
relationships

person (patient or client)
biopsychosocially, with his family

healthcare professional
Effective communication
Respectul care
Holistic perspective
Person-centered care
Empowerment
Family-centered
Interprofessional coordination
Interpersonal relationship
Cultural knowledge and skills
Social justice

Fig. 3.1 Collaborative relationship, naar: Lor et al. 2016. (beeldrechten: [rechten bij auteur], bestand:)

The relationship with the patient takes shape and content in the nursing process. The nursing process starts with the assessment, in which the patient history is the starting point. Subsequently, problems are identified, with which the nurse arrives at nursing diagnoses. The nursing process is followed by identifying the desired patient outcomes, health outcomes, where interventions are discussed with the patient based on short-term goals and a joint decision is made about which (nursing) interventions should be given priority.

In the implementation process of the intervention, as a nurse you continue to look for alignment and agreement and adjust diagnoses and interventions. Both diagnoses and interventions are subject to change as the patient's health status changes.

The final step is the evaluation in the nursing process, which evaluates whether the intended health effects have been achieved. But the evaluation phase also looks at whether the quality of life is assessed as good by the patient, and the focus is on patient satisfaction and how the patient has experienced the quality of care.

3.5   Conclusion

- Illness can be a life-changing experience, leaving patients feeling disconnected from themselves and their environment. Healthcare professionals must be mindful of this and work to provide relational care that takes into account the patient's unique needs and circumstances.
- By building a strong patient–nurse relationship and providing patient-specific, informative support, healthcare professionals can help patients navigate the challenges of illness and find a sense of agency and control in their lives. Ultimately, this is the foundation for effective care provision and better outcomes for patients.

Box 3.1 Mind-Map Impact of the Illness-Experience
Create a mind-map on the impact of the illness-experience on a person's perspective on life: how to recognize the impact of illness on the patient's life and how to help them learn to live with their health problem?

Box 3.2 Mind-Map Illness Always Raises Questions for the Patient
Create a mind-map on that Illness always raises questions for the patient. Create a mind-map focusing on the patient. Identify which common questions illness raises in the patient. Then select tools for nurses to deal with these.

Box 3.3 Mind-Map Important to Involve the Patient/Client in Their Care
Create a mind-map. It is important to involve the patient/client in the care they receive, because only then a person-centered care plan can be created. Create a mind-map putting the words "patient/client-centered care plan" in the middle. List the factors necessary to achieve a patient/client-centered care plan.

Next, circle what you expect from the patient/client themselves. Next, circle with a different color the factors where input is expected from the nursing professional.

Nursing and Patient History

4

4.1 Topic List: Care Should Be Individualized and Relational

1. Importance of individualized care: unique needs and concerns of patients about their illness.
2. Understanding personal living situation: culture, habits, health skills, preferences, activities of daily life, and personality of the patient.
3. Recognizing the patient's history: How illness can disrupt someone's life story and affect their self-image.
4. Resilience in dealing with illness: the challenges and coping strategies of patients.
5. Relational care: care from the point of view of the relationship with the patient.
6. Holistic view of humanity: all aspects of the biopsychosocial model in the relationship with the patient.
7. Importance of being seen, heard, listened to, and recognized as a person: enhancing patient satisfaction and quality of care.
8. Considering social networks of patients: the impact of family, work, associations, and social contacts on their health.
9. Care beyond disease recovery: patients remain connected to their own world and social environment.
10. Person-oriented care: relational connection with empathy and human friendliness as key characteristics of care.

4.2 Introduction

Providing personalized and individualized care is crucial for meeting the unique needs and concerns of patients and clients. It requires understanding their personal living situation, cultural background, health skills, preferences, and daily activities of patients, as well as their personality and history. Relational care is an approach that focuses on developing a relationship with the patient, involving all aspects of the biopsychosocial model, and recognizing the patient as a human being. It involves seeing the patient's illness as a disruption of their life story. Person-centered care and relational care is important in improving patient outcomes.

4.3   Outline

This chapter revolves around the importance of person-specific care and the exploration of a patient's unique needs and concerns about their illness. It emphasizes the need to understand the personal living situation, culture, habits, health skills, preferences, and activities of daily life of the patient. The chapter also discusses the importance of knowing the patient's history, including their work, social involvement, and medical history, to provide relational care. The focus is on providing care that is given with a view to relationships and ensuring that the patient remains connected to their own world. The topics highlight the importance of empathy and human friendliness in achieving the desired relational connection and providing person-oriented care. Overall, the chapter emphasize the importance of viewing the patient as a whole person and providing care that considers their social environment and personal history.

4.4   History of the Patient

Care should be individualized, and care should explore a patient's unique needs, as well as a patient's concerns about their illness. For this it is important that you get a picture of the personal living situation, together with the possibilities of a patient to make decisions and to have control over care (Suhonen et al. 2000). This personal life situation is about culture, habits, health skills, preferences, and activities of daily life and the patient's personality. It is about the patient's unique history (Morgan and Yoder 2012).

For relational care it is important to know the patient's history. His history takes the patient with him if he gets sick. Illness can disrupt someone's life story, especially in the case of a chronic illness. It thwarts one's expectations of life, the plans, and goals that one has in mind. Illness can affect one's self-image. For most people, vulnerability does not fit into the life plan, certainly not in the current times in which self-realization and autonomy occupy a central place. And then it suddenly turns out that health is not self-evident, that your body or mind is faltering and does not do what you want. Instead of a body and/or mind you have that is the vehicle of your plans for this life, you are confronted with a body that plans its own plan. It takes a lot of resilience to deal with this.

Providing relational care is about care that is provided from the point of view of the relationship with the patient (Baart 2018).

Relational care is about care that is provided as a relationship (Baart 2018). It is important that the nursing professional sees the patient as a human being, from a holistic view of humanity and involves all aspects of the biopsychosocial model in that relationship with the patient. A patient or client wants to be seen, heard, listened to and recognized as a person. Then there can be good care.

Relational care is about care that is provided in relationships (Baart 2018).

Every patient is a person with a history. Knowing the history of a patient or client is important to understand the person, and depending on their age, it will be a short of longer history that has an impact on the illness experience. This person is a human being with a family and work history, and possibly a medical history. It is a person with a past of social involvement, for example, in associations, and social contacts. Virtually every patient or client is surrounded by other people, by relatives. Sometimes this involves extensive social networks, sometimes a narrow network with only contact with neighbors (Fig. 4.1).

Providing relational care is about care provided by relationships, but also about care that is given with a view on relationships (Baart 2018). This means that the care is not only focused on recovering from the disease. It is about ensuring that the

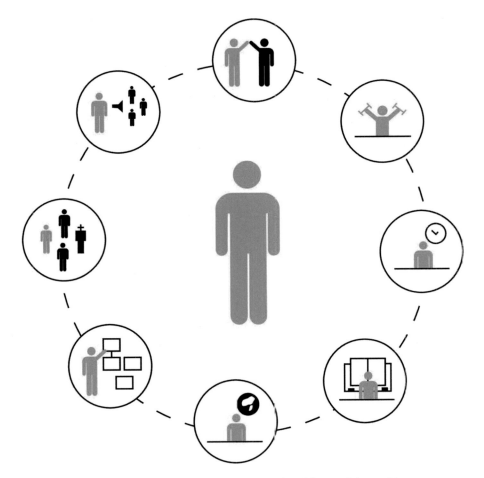

Fig. 4.1 Social networks of patients. (beeldrechten: [rechten bij auteur], bestand:)

patient remains connected to his own world. This means that the care is not only aimed at the patient as a whole, but that his social environment must also be involved and remain involved. This social world consists of the family or household to which someone belongs, the work situation, the sports club, and so on.

By providing care with a view to the patient's environment, you avoid someone from becoming disconnected from their environment. Regaining the living environment when contact has been broken due to the illness is a difficult process for patients. Maintaining contact with the social environment makes it easier for the patient to continue his life in the circumstances that the patient finds most comfortable.

Person-oriented care means that the patient experiences a relational connection with the nurse. The nurse maintains a relationship with the patient in which the keynote consists of empathy and human friendliness. This is because empathy is an important characteristic of human-friendly care and is essential to achieve the desired relational connection.

4.5   Conclusion

Providing person-centered and relational care is essential for improving patient outcomes. Understanding the patient's personal living situation, cultural background, and history can help healthcare providers provide individualized care that meets the unique needs and concerns of patients. The relational care approach focuses on developing a relationship with the patient, involving all aspects of the biopsychosocial model, and recognizing the patient as a human being. By maintaining a connection with the patient's social environment, healthcare providers can help patients stay connected to their world and regain their living environment when contact has been broken due to illness. Empathy and human friendliness are essential characteristics of relational care that can help healthcare providers achieve the desired relational connection with patients.

Box 4.1 Mind-Map Exploring a Patient's Unique Needs
Create a mind-map on the need for care that explores a patient's unique needs and concerns about their illness. What needs to be understood in a patient's personal living situation, culture, habits, health skills, preferences, and activities of daily life, along with their personality and history, to provide better care?

Box 4.2 Mind-Map Importance of Empathy and Human Friendliness
Create a mind-map: the importance of empathy and human friendliness in person-oriented care. What are crucial characteristic of human-friendly care essential for achieving the desired relational connection between the healthcare provider and the patient?

Nursing and ICF from the Perspective of Health

5

5.1 Topic List

1. In the ICF (International Classification of Functioning, Disability and Health), Health Is Also Viewed from the Biopsychosocial Model.
2. Overview of the International Classification of Functioning, Disability and Health (ICF) and its significance for nursing professionals.
3. Understanding health as viewed in the ICF the biopsychosocial model.
4. Importance of optimizing health status and identifying health risks in nursing practice.
5. Placing the patient's health status in the context of daily functioning and social functioning in the ICF.
6. Perceived quality of life as an important patient outcome for nursing care.
7. Impact of chronic health problems and multimorbidity on perceived quality of life.
8. Definition of health in the ICF and its relationship with the World Health Organization's definition of health.
9. Six dimensions of health in the ICF: physical, mental, spiritual/existential, social, quality of life, and general daily life skills.
10. Resilience and self-management as key aspects of positive health in the ICF.
11. Healthy people 2020 report by WHO and its emphasis on a broader context of health, including social and environmental factors.
12. Health promotion and creating a conducive social and physical environment for health in the ICF.
13. Shifting the focus of care from disease to health in the ICF and its implications for nursing practice.

5.2   Introduction

The International Classification of Functioning, Disability and Health (ICF) views health from a biopsychosocial perspective. It places the patient's health condition in the context of their daily functioning and social environment, with the aim of optimizing their health status and identifying health risks that could lead to a deterioration in their health. As nursing professionals, understanding the ICF is crucial because it highlights the relationship between health status and impairments, limitations, and disabilities. Furthermore, optimizing the perceived quality of life is a key outcome for care, especially when patients experience reduced quality of life due to chronic health conditions or multimorbidity.

5.3   Outline

This chapter discusses the International Classification of Functioning, Disability and Health (ICF) , which provides a biopsychosocial model to view health. Nurses are encouraged to optimize health status and identify health risks that could lead to a decline in health status. The ICF considers a patient's health status in the context of their daily functioning, with an emphasis on social functioning. The ICF also acknowledges that disruptions in health status can lead to impairments, limitations, and disabilities.

The chapter highlights the importance of improving the perceived quality of life as a way to optimize patients' health status. Quality of life is measured based on physical, psychological, and social functioning, and it is subjectively evaluated by patients. This assessment provides nurses with valuable information and is a significant outcome of care.

The ICF and the World Health Organization (WHO) define health as the ability to adapt and self-manage in the face of physical, emotional, and social challenges. Additionally, the WHO emphasizes that health is a resource for everyday life that emphasizes social and personal resources as well as physical capabilities.

It is essential to consider social and environmental factors that influence people's health status when looking at health in a broader context. The goal of Healthy People 2020 is to create a society in which all people live long and healthy lives. Health promotion is encouraged by developing and stimulating a healthy lifestyle for people of all ages. The focus of care has shifted from disease treatment to expanding health.

5.4   ICF's Perspective on Health

In the ICF (International Classification of Functioning, Disability and Health), health is also viewed from the biopsychosocial model. The patient's health condition is the starting point in the ICF (Fig. 5.1). Nurses should focus on optimizing health status and identifying health risks that could lead to a deterioration in health status. The model places the patient's health status in the context of his daily functioning, with an eye for a person's social functioning. The ICF is important for nursing

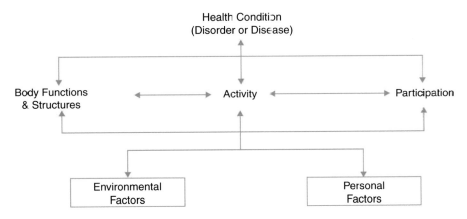

Fig. 5.1 The interaction between different aspects of health status and external and personal factors. (Source: ICF. beeldrechten: [rechten bij auteur], bestand:)

professionals because it shows that disturbances in the patient's health status can lead to impairments, limitations, and disabilities.

When we as nurses talk about optimizing the health status of patients, it is often about improving the perceived quality of life. Quality of life is the functioning of people on a physical, psychological, and social level and the assessment that people themselves give to this. People, therefore, judge their own health themselves and this is always a subjective assessment.

This assessment of perceived quality of life gives nursing professionals valuable information and is significant as a patient outcome for care. When people get sick, they often experience a reduced quality of life. If people have a chronic health problem or if there is multimorbidity, the perceived quality of life is often judged even more unfavorably.

Continuing with the ICF, health is seen as:

> … the ability of people to adapt and self-manage in the face of physical, emotional and social challenges of life. Being healthy means being able to adapt to disturbances, being resilient, being able to maintain or regain a balance physically, mentally and socially. (Source: Huber and Staps 2016). In this definition, positive health is referred to. It focuses on six dimensions of health: physical, mental, spiritual/existential, and social dimensions of health, quality of life, and general daily life skills. The emphasis is on people's resilience and their ability to self-manage (Huber and Staps 2016).

The definition of the ICF derives from the World Health Organization's (World Health Organization;, WHO) definition of health:

> Health is […] enabling people to increase control over and to improve their health. (Bron: WHO 1986)

And:

> Health is a resource for everyday life, not the object of living. It is a positive concept emphasizing social and personal resources as well as physical capabilities. (Bron: WHO 1999)

In its Healthy people 2020 report, WHO emphasizes the importance of looking at health in a broader context, with an emphasis on the influence that social and environmental factors have on people's health status. The goal of Healthy people 2020 is "a society in which all people live long, healthy lives."

Improving health status by expanding health is about:

- preventing disease;
- avoiding health inequalities, and
- improving people's health.

It is also about creating a social and physical environment that is conducive to health. The emphasis is on health promotion by developing and stimulating a healthy lifestyle for people in all age groups (www.healthypeople.gov). The point of departure for care is no longer disease but is aimed at (expanding) health.

5.5   Conclusion

- The ICF definition of health emphasizes the ability of individuals to adapt and self-manage physical, emotional, and social challenges of life. It also stresses the importance of positive health, which includes six dimensions of health: physical, mental, spiritual/existential, social, quality of life, and daily life skills.
- The WHO's Healthy People 2020 report emphasizes the importance of looking at health in a broader context and promoting health by developing and stimulating a healthy lifestyle for all age groups.
- As healthcare professionals, nurses have an important role in expanding health by preventing diseases, avoiding health inequalities, and improving the overall health of their patients.
- By adopting a biopsychosocial approach and utilizing the ICF, nurses can optimize their patients' health status and promote positive health outcomes.

> **Box 5.1 Mind-Map Using ICF to Optimize a patient's Health Status**
> Create a mind-map on how the different components of the ICF model can be used to optimize a patient's health status by identifying health risks that could lead to impairments, limitations, and disabilities. Choose a specific case or patient−/client group and specify the component of the ICF.

> **Box 5.2 Mind-Map Perceived Quality of Life as a Patient Outcome**
> Create a mind-map on perceived Quality of Life as a patient outcome for care. How can a patient's assessment of their own health, provide valuable information for you as a nursing professional? And for people having chronic health problems or multimorbidity, is this assessment even more important?

Box 5.3 Mind-Map Expanding Health, the Importance of Prevention
Create a mind-map on expanding health. Point out the importance of preventing disease, avoiding health inequalities, and improving people's health. Make it applicable for all age groups.

Box 5.4 Mind-Map All People Live Long, Healthy Lives
Create a mind-map on the goal of Healthy people 2020, point out how to create a society in which all people live long, healthy lives, and point out how nursing care can play a role in achieving this goal.

Nursing and (Professional) Health Perception

6

6.1 Topic List

1. Understanding that each patient has their own views on health.
2. Recognizing that your own views on health may differ from those of your patients.
3. Being aware that your views on health are shaped by education and professional experience.
4. Avoiding imposing your own views on health on the patient.
5. Understanding that patients may need good reasons to change their health behaviors.
6. Recognizing that patients may consider taking action on their health problems based on the severity of symptoms, perceived solvability, and potential reduction of symptoms.
7. Acknowledging that patients' knowledge about their health problem may have limited influence on their health behavior.
8. Understanding that patients differ in their ability to communicate effectively and share their feelings, preferences, and concerns.
9. Taking into account patients' personal characteristics, education level, and culture in communication and care.
10. Paying attention, offering relevant information, and actively listening to help patients feel seen and valued.
11. Creating a safe and accepting environment for patients to cooperate in the care and treatment process.

© The Author(s), under exclusive license to Springer Nature
Switzerland AG 2023
B. Sassen, *Improving Person-Centered Innovation of Nursing Care*,
https://doi.org/10.1007/978-3-031-35048-1_6

6.2   Introduction

Healthcare providers often have their own views and beliefs about what constitutes good health, based on their education and experience. However, it is important for them to recognize that their patients may have different beliefs about their own health. It is not appropriate for healthcare providers to impose their own beliefs on their patients or to assume that the patient's starting point is the same as their own. Effective communication and understanding are key to establishing a successful partnership between healthcare providers and patients.

6.3   Outline

This chapter emphasizes the importance of recognizing and respecting the individual views and beliefs that patients have regarding their own health. The author notes that healthcare providers may have different views on health, but it is important not to impose these views on the patient or take them for granted when providing care and treatment. Patients may need good reasons to make changes to their health behaviors, such as when they experience severe symptoms or believe that a commitment to treatment can lead to a reduction in symptoms. However, the patient's knowledge about their health problem has only a limited influence on their behavior. This chapter discusses that patients differ in their ability to effectively communicate their feelings, preferences, and concerns, and these differences can arise from their personal characteristics, education level, and culture. Healthcare providers can support patients by actively listening, offering relevant information, and taking into account their personal knowledge and background.

6.4   Health Perceptions Differ

Each patient has his own views about his health. Your own views on health often cannot and often will not coincide with the views on health of your patients. Your health views are shaped by your education and professional experience. Your own health views should not be imposed on the patient. Nor should these views on health be taken for granted as the starting point for care and treatment.

Patients (because of their own health views) need good reasons to behave differently, in a healthier way. It is often the case that patients will consider getting started with their health (problems) themselves ...:

- if the symptoms of their disease are experienced as (very) severe.
- if the symptoms are acute, but seem to be solvable; and
- if a certain commitment can lead to a perceptible reduction of symptoms.
- The knowledge a patient has about his health problem has only a very limited influence on the patient's health behavior.

Patients differ in their ability to communicate effectively, and to effectively share their feelings, preferences, and concerns (Epstein and Street 2011). These differences between people arise from the patient's views on health, but also from personal characteristics, education level, and culture. By paying attention, offering relevant information and listening actively, you help the patient to feel seen. You take the personal knowledge and background of each patient into account. If the patient feels safe, accepted, and valued by healthcare professionals, it is easier for the patient to cooperate in the care treatment process (Arnold and Underman Boggs 2020).

6.5   Conclusion

- Each patient has their own unique views and beliefs about their health, and it is important for healthcare providers to recognize and respect these differences.
- Patients require good reasons to make changes to their health behaviors, and healthcare providers can support them by providing relevant, person-specific health-education, listening actively, and taking into account their personal knowledge and background.
- By establishing a partnership based on understanding and mutual respect, healthcare providers can work together with their patients to achieve better health outcomes.

> **Box 6.1 Mind-Map Professionals' Personal Health Views**
> Create a mind-map: How do healthcare professionals' personal health views influence the care and treatment they provide? What can be done to ensure that healthcare professionals are aware of their biases and do not impose their views on patients?

> **Box 6.2 Mind-Map Different Communication Styles**
> Create a mind-map: How can healthcare professionals effectively communicate with patients who have different communication styles, backgrounds, and levels of health literacy? What strategies can be used to ensure that patients feel comfortable and confident in discussing their health concerns and needs?

Nursing and General and Mental Health Care

7

7.1 Topic List

1. The biopsychosocial model as a starting point in patient care.
2. The dichotomy between mental health care and general health care.
3. Comorbidity of physical and mental health problems in patients.
4. Challenges in addressing physical health in mental health care.
5. Unfavorable life expectancy and lifestyle in patients with mental health problems.
6. Shortcomings in the integration of physical and mental health care.
7. Moving towards personalized healthcare in mental health and general health care.
8. Patient perception of illness and the need for understanding.
9. Nurse's role in gaining insight into patient's perception of illness.
10. Perceived susceptibility, severity, and control in patient's experience of illness.

7.2 Introduction

In healthcare, the division between mental and physical health care often results in patients receiving fragmented and inconsistent care. Mental health problems are primarily treated by mental health facilities, while general health problems are treated by medical facilities. However, this dichotomy often fails to address the coexistence of physical and mental health problems in patients or clients. This chapter explores the importance of the biopsychosocial model and the need to integrate mental and physical health care to meet the individual needs of patients.

© The Author(s), under exclusive license to Springer Nature
Switzerland AG 2023
B. Sassen, *Improving Person-Centered Innovation of Nursing Care*,
https://doi.org/10.1007/978-3-031-35048-1_7

7.3   Outline

This chapter discusses the need for healthcare professionals to consider both the physical and mental health of patients, as well as the shortcomings in the current division between mental and general health care. The importance of taking patient needs and individuality into account is emphasized, along with the need for integrated care and personalized healthcare. This chapter also discusses the patient's perception of illness and the importance of understanding their perceptions and specific patient needs in order to provide effective care. Finally, the World Health Organization's framework for understanding a patient's vulnerability to illness, perceived severity of illness, and control over their health and behaviors is mentioned as a guide for healthcare professionals.

7.4   Integrating General and Mental Healthcare

If we start from the biopsychosocial model and always take this as a starting point in the relationship with the patient, then an important starting point is that we look at both the physical and mental health of patients. In healthcare, however, there is a division between the different disciplines: When we look at the organization of healthcare, we see healthcare facilities that deal with mental, psychological health problems; and on the other hand, health care facilities that focus on general, medical, physical health problems. Reasoned from the needs of patients and clients, this dichotomy is often not easy to handle.

From the past, attention in mental health care is almost exclusively focused on mental health problems and that in general health care attention is focused on physical health problems. In doing so, many common cases in which this dichotomy is at odds are ignored. For example, a person with depressive symptoms is being treated by mental health care, but also suffers from high blood pressure, a high blood cholesterol level and increasingly has problems with his eyes. For example, a person with renal impairment who is on dialysis due to the insufficient functioning of his kidneys feels anxious and depressed due to the chronicity of his health problem. Considering patient needs as the starting point of care and treatment, health care professionals should continually consider both physical and mental patient needs, patient problems and health problems. This would do justice to the individuality of each patient and to the diversity among people.

The treatment paradigm in mental health care has mainly changed as a result of pharmacological developments. Due to changes in medication, the roles of healthcare professionals have changed (Thompson and McCabe 2012).

A study shows that people in treatment for psychiatric health problems, the mental health problem coexists with physical health problems. People with a psychiatric illness are twice as likely to also have physical health problems compared to the general population without psychiatric health problems. Comorbidity is more often not diagnosed in people with psychiatric health problems, and the focus on prevention is minimal (Happell et al. 2012).

People with psychiatric health problems also more often have an unfavorable life expectancy, due to both an unfavorable lifestyle and the side effects of antipsychotics. Furthermore, in patients with unstable mental status, with high levels of psychotic symptoms or depression, physical symptoms, and health problems appear to be overlooked. In this patient population, the emphasis is strongly on risk management, for the patient himself and for others, as a result of which care providers ignore the patient's (unhealthy) lifestyle and physical health problems (Bradshaw and Pedley 2012).

The division between mental health and general health care can be seen as a shortcoming in the health care system as a whole. In mental health care, physical health did not appear to be a priority in daily care. The provision of care was ad hoc, inconsistent, and fragmented (Happell et al 2012). Prevention and lifestyle management, such as with regard to side effects of drugs and implications of drug use on daily life, received little attention. An example is sexual problems that may arise as a result of the use of psychotropic medication, resulting in a relapse. Another problem is weight gain with the use of antipsychotic medication (Happell et al. 2012).

Integrating health services would be in line with the holistic view and the biopsychosocial approach. If there is integrated care, the physical problems of people in care because of psychological or psychiatric health problems can be integrated into the care and treatment they receive in mental health care. Conversely, psychological problems can be included in the care and treatment of patients with physical problems in regular care.

Another fact is that we want to move towards personalized healthcare, care tailored to the patient's specific individual care needs. This is becoming the standard for mental health care, but also in general health care (Vlek et al. 2013).

Tailoring the care to the personal care needs of the patient requires insight into the patient's perception of illness. When people become ill, we often see that the patient is looking for an answer to the question: 'Why me? Why do I get this disease?' Finding explanations enables the patient to communicate about his disease, to choose treatment options and to interpret the symptoms. The answers to this essential question make the patient better understand his own illness.

When sick, the patient becomes aware that his body (physical) or mind (psyche) has failed him. Illness fuels the need to understand physical or psychological processes. In the event of illness, people assess their physical and mental condition as "expectable," as "worrying" or as "requiring treatment and care." Every human being needs an expectation of the future that one experiences as meaningful. Human beings have a need to understand themselves and to be understood by others.

The nurse in both general and mental health care wants to gain insight into how the patient:

- perceives his vulnerability to the illness (perceived susceptibility to illness);
- how serious and threatening the illness is experienced by the patient (perceived severity of illness); and
- the extent in which the patient experiences having control over his illness, his own health, and health behaviors (WHO 2003).

7.5   Conclusion

- The integration of mental and physical health care is crucial to address the coexistence of physical and mental health problems in patients and clients.
- The biopsychosocial model provides a holistic approach to patient care, which focuses on physical, psychological, and social factors. Healthcare providers need to be aware of the prevalence of comorbidity in mental health patients and prioritize prevention and lifestyle management to improve patient outcomes.
- Tailoring care to the individual needs of patients requires insight into their perception of illness, which can help them understand their illness and choose appropriate treatment options.
- By integrating mental and physical health care, we can ensure that patients receive comprehensive and individualized, person-centered care that meets their needs.

Box 7.1 Mind-Map Dichotomy as Challenges the Integrated Care
Create a mind-map. The dichotomy between mental health care and general health care poses challenges the integrated care of patients who have comorbid physical and mental health problems.

How can health care professionals address this shortcoming in the health care system to provide holistic care that meets the individual needs of patients?

Box 7.2 Mind-Map Recognize and Integrate
Create a mind-map. In general health care, mental and psychiatric health problems occur in about one in every four patients.

This figure does not include common complaints (such as anxiety, sleep problems, dejection, and lethargy).

Start from the field of care (general or mental health) where your own interest lies. Make a mind map of how to recognize and integrate mental health problems into care from your chosen field of care (e.g., general health care). Suppose you work in mental health care; how can you recognize and integrate physical health problems into care.

Nursing and Presence Approach

8

8.1 Topic-List for "The Presence Approach in Patient Care"

1. Introduction to the Presence Approach: Definition and Principles.
2. Importance of Building a Relationship of Trust with Patients.
3. Application of the presence Approach in Care for People who are Difficult to Reach.
4. Overcoming Prejudice in Patient Care: A Positive and Respectful Approach.
5. Care-Ethical Perspective of the Presence Approach.
6. Avoiding Dominance of Professional Thinking in Patient Care.
7. Patient-Centered Care: Focusing on Unique Biopsychosocial Needs.
8. Holistic View of Patients as Biopsychosocial Units in Care.
9. Starting with Patient's Wishes and Expectations in Care Planning.
10. Identifying Patient Needs and Aligning Care and Treatment Offer.
11. Challenging Traditional Thinking in Healthcare: A Turnaround in Patient-Centered Care.
12. Benefits of a Relationship of Trust in Caring for Patients with Complex Care Questions or Isolated Lives.

8.2 Introduction

The presence approach is a care-ethical way of thinking that focuses on building a relationship of trust between the healthcare professional and the patient. It is particularly suitable for patients who are difficult to reach or have complex care needs. The approach involves treating the patient without prejudice, with a positive and respectful attitude, and learning to speak each other's language. This approach recognizes the importance of seeing the patient as a unique individual with biopsychosocial needs. In this way, care and treatment are tailored to the patient's specific situation, increasing the chance of meeting their needs.

© The Author(s), under exclusive license to Springer Nature Switzerland AG 2023
B. Sassen, *Improving Person-Centered Innovation of Nursing Care*,
https://doi.org/10.1007/978-3-031-35048-1_8

8.3   Outline

This chapter describes the "presence approach" in healthcare, which involves establishing a relationship of trust with the patient and treating them without prejudice, even if they deviate from the norm. The approach is appropriate for people who are difficult to reach or have complex care questions. We discuss that this is a care-ethical way of thinking that emphasizes the importance of learning to speak each other's language. We also discuss the importance of not allowing professional thinking to dominate appropriate care and treatment, and how good care should be determined by what the patient needs, with their unique biopsychosocial needs taken into account. Finally, the topic emphasizes that starting from a relationship of trust makes it easier to connect with people who are more difficult to reach or have complex care questions. This requires a turnaround in the thinking of healthcare professionals about illness and health, with patient needs taking center stage.

8.4   Being Present

The presence approach is about establishing a relationship with the patient and building a relationship of trust. The aim is for the patient to experience that he is being seen. The presence approach is appropriate for people who are more difficult to reach or who have complex care questions. Think of people who live very isolated lives from society. The basic principle is that the patient is treated without prejudice, even if someone deviates from the norm. The approach towards the patient is a positive, respectful approach. The presence approach is a care-ethical way of thinking, where it is about learning to speak each other's language.

We should not allow the dominance of professional thinking to get in the way of appropriate care and treatment. What constitutes good care should not be determined by all kinds of rules. But good care is above all what a patient of client needs. Baart (2018) refers to this as "continuing to see the good." Good care would consist of what the unique patient needs, with his unique biopsychosocial needs.

When we think from a holistic view of man and approach the patient as a biopsychosocial unit, the needs of the patient are the starting point of care (Fig. 8.1). This starts with making an inventory of the patient's wishes and expectations together with the patient. This basis significantly increases the chance that the care and treatment offer is in line with the patient's (health) situation.

The starting point is then which patient needs have I identified together with the patient and which care and treatment offer fits in with this. What are the patient's needs and what is most appropriate to deal with the patient's illness and health situation? This thinking based on patient needs is new and requires a turnaround (switch) in the thinking of health care professionals about illness and health.

Starting from a relationship of trust makes it easier to connect with people who are more difficult to reach or have more complex care questions.

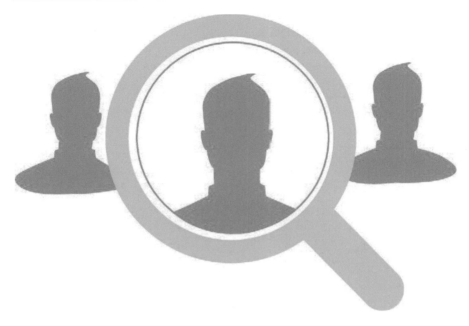

Fig. 8.1 Zooming in on patient needs. (beeldrechten: [rechten bij auteur], bestand:)

8.5   Conclusion

- The presence approach is a significant shift in the way healthcare professionals think about care and treatment. It recognizes the importance of building a relationship of trust and treating the patient with respect and without prejudice.
- By focusing on the patient's unique needs and situation, care and treatment can be tailored to fit the patient, increasing the likelihood of successful outcomes.
- It is essential that healthcare professionals prioritize the patient's needs and work towards a holistic view of the patient as a biopsychosocial unit to provide appropriate care and treatment.
- Ultimately, the presence approach is about seeing the good in every patient and ensuring that their care is centered around their needs.

Box 8.1 Mind-Map Establishing a Relationship of Trust
Create a mind-map on the importance of establishing a relationship of trust with patients. The presence approach emphasizes the need for healthcare professionals to establish a relationship of trust with their patients. This is especially important for people who are more difficult to reach or who have complex care questions, such as those who live very isolated lives from society.

How can healthcare professionals build and maintain trust with their patients?

What are some of the barriers that can prevent trust from developing?

Box 8.2 Mind-Map Importance Presence Approach

Create a mind-map on the importance of patient-centered care: The presence approach emphasizes the importance of focusing on the needs of the patient and providing care that is tailored to their unique biopsychosocial needs. This requires healthcare professionals to take a holistic view of the patient and to work in partnership with them to develop a care plan that is appropriate to their individual needs.

Point out: what are the benefits of a patient-centered approach to care?

How can healthcare professionals ensure that their care is truly patient-centered? Specify for all benefits.

Box 8.3 Mind-Map Challenges Presence Approach

Create a mind-map on the challenges of shifting towards a patient-centered approach. The presence approach represents a shift in the way that healthcare professionals think about illness and health. It requires them to move away from a dominant professional perspective and to focus on the needs of the patient. However, making this shift can be challenging, as it requires healthcare professionals to unlearn old habits and to adopt new ways of working.

Point out: what are some of the challenges that healthcare professionals may face in adopting a patient-centered approach?

How can they be handled?

Nursing and the Provision of Care and Treatment

9

9.1 Topic List

1. Our Current Health Care System Is Strongly Organized in Terms of Care and Treatment.
2. Medical-dominated contacts in healthcare: one-way communication and lack of patient participation.
3. Shift towards person-centered care: focusing on the patient's individual needs, preferences, and well-being.
4. Changing role of healthcare professionals: from authoritarian to partnership-focused relationships with patients.
5. Importance of empathetic and exploratory approach by nurses: Understanding the patient's biopsychosocial situation and addressing their concerns.
6. Challenges in thinking outside the range of care and treatment: Overcoming professional frameworks and offering patient-centered care.
7. Non-judgmental approach towards patients: Avoiding blame and focusing on solutions.
8. Patient's perspective in healthcare: Moving away from disease-focused care to holistic care considering the patient's overall health, psychological well-being, and social circumstances.
9. Collaborative decision-making: Involving patients in the care planning process and determining care options together.
10. Addressing delayed healthcare-seeking behavior: Understanding patients' reasons for delay and offering appropriate solutions.
11. Importance of professionalism and expertise in providing patient-centered care: Balancing clinical knowledge with patient needs for optimal care.

B. Sassen, *Improving Person-Centered Innovation of Nursing Care*, https://doi.org/10.1007/978-3-031-35048-1_9

9.2   Introduction

Our current healthcare system is heavily focused on diagnosis, referral, and specific treatments tailored to the diagnosed disease. However, from the patient's perspective, the starting point should be their individual and specific patient needs, encompassing their medical, psychological, and social circumstances. Healthcare professionals have been trained to provide care and treatment based on the patient's health complaint, but a person-centered perspective is necessary to truly meet the patient's needs. This approach involves exploring the patient's concerns and needs, so that the patient is seen and feels seen.

9.3   Outline

This chapter discusses the importance of prioritizing the needs of the patient in nursing care. It emphasizes that the approach should not only rely on rules, guidelines, and protocols, but rather on what the patient requires. The passage highlights the importance of considering the patient's specific health issues, social context, and emotional state. Discussed is that an empathetic and exploratory approach is crucial to ensure the patient feels seen and heard. Additionally, it is discussed that it may be a challenge to think beyond the scope of care and treatment and the responsibility of healthcare professionals to provide non-judgmental care and align with the patient's needs. Overall, the passage emphasizes the importance of responding to the patient's needs with expertise and professionalism to provide patient-centered care.

9.4   Combining Perspectives

Our current health care system is strongly organized in terms of care and treatment. The way healthcare is organized now, is that the patient is diagnosed with a certain disease and given a referral to a specific healthcare provider. This healthcare professional offers a specific treatment that is tailored to the diagnosed disease.

Nothing to worry about, you might think, after all, that's what the patient is there for. But here is more to it. From the patient's point of view, the starting point is his individual and specific patient needs: his ideas and wishes about what best suits his medical and biological situation, his psychological health and his social circumstances.

Healthcare professionals are trained to master a specific healthcare offering and to provide their care and treatment from there. They have learned to think in terms of the patient's health complaint and to respond to this with a specific care and treatment offer. In short: the complaint or health problem of the patient or client, requires a solution from the healthcare professional. This solution is sought from the palette of available interventions that a specific healthcare professional has at his disposal. The care and treatment on offer therefore determines the care and treatment that is used.

However, it requires a different view of care and treatment if, as a professional, you look at the wishes and needs of the patient from a person-centered perspective. This instead of "sticking" the care and treatment offerings to the patient (Fig. 9.1).

That patients are asked to be more active in contacting and entering into a relationship with nurses and other healthcare professionals is in contrast to the medical-dominated contacts that have long defined healthcare. In the medically-dominated contacts, there was little or no room for the patient to take an active role and to indicate his patient needs. The professional "knew" the solution to the patient's problem, and this medical dominance left its mark on the doctor–patient relationship. Communication was often very much one-way.

Nowadays, health professionals adapt their actions not only to the patient's problem but also to their biopsychosocial situation. The patient's needs are explored together, and the plan "how to handle this" is determined collaboratively. There is no longer one-way communication. Healthcare professionals have long derived their strength from the authoritarian role but have now transformed their role into a partnership-focused relationship. An empathetic attitude and a focus on cooperation within a friendly relationship are at the core (Epstein and Street 2011).

Taking this as a starting point as a nurse makes it easier to do the right thing for the patient. This nursing action would then not only arise from rules, guidelines, and protocols, but would be based on the question: "What does this patient need?".

We start from the needs of the patient or client. We look at their patient needs and take into account the patient's specific (chronic) health problem. We make an inventory of which disorders, limitations, and disabilities have arisen and how these

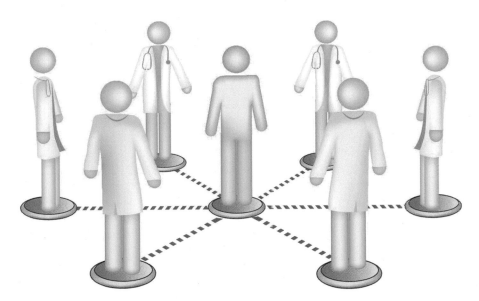

Fig. 9.1 Person-centered care. (beeldrechten: [rechten bij auteur], bestand:)

affect the health status of the patient. We look at the context in which the patient lives, what his social situation looks like. But above all we look at the patient's well-being: how does he feel? How is the patient doing? Is he nervous or even scared? Is he depressed and showing little emotion? The nurse should approach the patient with an empathetic, exploratory view. Always starting to explore, exploring the concerns, so that the patient is seen and feels seen.

The professional practice of nurses does not make thinking outside the range of care and treatment easy. Every healthcare professional works from his own framework and offers care based on his own professional responsibility. Besides always starting from exploring, exploring his needs, you help the patient by acting non-judgmentally. Don't say "you've been walking around with that for too long, why you didn't come sooner," but present a solution. The patient usually knows that he has waited "too long." Your approach should align with the patient's starting point, i.e., patient needs, and should be responded to with expertise and professionalism.

9.5   Conclusion

- Healthcare professionals need to shift their focus from solely providing care and treatment to meeting the individual needs of each patient.
- This person-centered approach involves exploring the patient's concerns and needs, listening to their opinions and views, and providing care based on their specific situation.
- It is important to approach each patient with empathy and non-judgmental attitudes, in order to provide care that is responsive and professional.
- By doing so, we can ensure that our healthcare system is not just focused on diagnoses and treatments, but on meeting the needs of each patient, ultimately improving their overall well-being and perceived quality of life.

Box 9.1 Mind-Map Importance of Person-Centered Care
Create a mind-map on the importance of person-centered care in healthcare. The current healthcare system is strongly organized in terms of care and treatment, but there is a growing need to shift towards person-centered care.

Healthcare professionals are often trained to think in terms of specific treatments and interventions.

Point out why it can be difficult to shift towards a more holistic and collaborative approach. Make an inventory of factors.

And additionally, healthcare organizations may need to restructure their systems and processes to support person-centered care. Make an inventory how to "handle" the factors.

Box 9.2 Mind-Map a Shift in Mindset
Create a mind-map: Nurses can play a key role in delivering person-centered care, as they are often the healthcare professionals who have the most direct and frequent contact with patients.

Point out: what do you/nursing professionals need to make a shift in mindset from a focus on tasks and procedures to a focus on the patient's needs and well-being?

And point out, how can nursing professionals bridge the gap between the patient and other healthcare professionals, ensuring that the patient's needs are being addressed in a coordinated and comprehensive manner?

Box 9.3 Mind-Map Redefine This Care Offer
Create a mind map of your own nursing care offerings for the patient group(s) you see most often. For example, these might be people with depressive symptoms or patients with cardiovascular disease.

Redefine this care offer from a patient perspective and needs, that is, formulate from the patient needs each element of the care offer you listed.

Box 9.4 Mind-Map Specific Care Offerings
Create a mind map for a patient group, or better; for a specific patient. For example, think back to the last patient who impressed you or the last to whom you provided care.

Create the mind map for: "What does this patient need?" and make it clear how you then accomplish that with specific care offerings.

Nursing and Vulnerable People

10

10.1 Topic List: Vulnerable Patients and Health Inequalities

1. Exploring groups of people who are more vulnerable than others due to health problems or life adversities.
2. Health literacy and vulnerability in patients, including difficulties in understanding health information and applying it in their own situation.
3. Challenges in communication: vulnerable patients, such as those with limited health skills, fluency issues, cognitive limitations, or social disadvantages, face challenges in understanding and participating in their own care.
4. Providing relational care for vulnerable patients, where the relationship with healthcare professionals plays a crucial role in their care.
5. Disparities in care: disconnect between patient satisfaction with care and incomplete understanding and participation in care, particularly in vulnerable populations.
6. Socio-economic factors: impact of socio-economic disadvantages on health inequalities and the need for nursing support and advocacy for patients and families in such situations.
7. Equity in health: importance of assessing patient needs with a focus on improving equity in health and addressing health inequalities.
8. Nursing interventions: role of nurses in identifying and intervening appropriately to minimize health inequalities and improve the quality of life and care for vulnerable patients.

10.2 Introduction

Vulnerable patients are a group that needs special attention from healthcare professionals. These patients are often more susceptible to health problems and also experience difficulties in functioning properly in society. Limited health literacy is often

B. Sassen, *Improving Person-Centered Innovation of Nursing Care*, https://doi.org/10.1007/978-3-031-35048-1_10

seen as a common issue among vulnerable patients, which makes it more challenging for them to understand health-related information. In this context, nurses play a crucial role in providing adequate care to this group of patients, ensuring that they communicate in a way that is easily understandable and addressing their specific patient needs.

10.3 Outline

This chapter discusses the concept of vulnerable patients, who are more susceptible to health problems and difficulties in functioning properly in society. Additionally, vulnerable patients often have less optimal health literacy, meaning that they may struggle to understand information about their own health, struggle to handle self-management or lifestyle changes, and difficulties in making informed health-related decisions. This chapter discusses that nurses should pay attention to this group of people and provide relational care to help them understand their health situation and make informed decisions. This specifically for people with limited health skills, those for whom speaking fluently is a problem, those with cognitive limitations, and those with social disadvantages are at the greatest risk of experiencing a disconnect between patient satisfaction with care and incomplete understanding and participation in care. Nurses should be aware of these patients' specific needs and work to improve equity in health and provide appropriate care to minimize health inequalities.

10.4 Needs of Vulnerable People

There are groups of people who are more vulnerable than other groups of patients. This vulnerability can be about an extra vulnerability to health problems, but more often it is about a vulnerability to life's adversities. Vulnerable patients are more often ill and due to their health problems, also more often experience difficulties in functioning in society. Vulnerable patients are also more likely to have less optimal health literacy skills. Health skills are the skills you need to find your way in the healthcare system as a patient. For example, the ability to read a package leaflet, to understand the conversation with the nurse properly or to be able to make a subsequent appointment. Nurses should pay attention to this group of people.

Health literacy is often associated with low literacy. Nursing professionals should anticipate that it may be more difficult for this group of people to properly understand information about their own (health) situation. The switch between hearing general information and applying it in their own specific (health) situation is also experienced as more complex by this group. Nurses should certainly, in the case of health-related decisions, ensure that they communicate with vulnerable patients in a way that makes it possible for them to discuss together what their wishes and patient needs are. And it is always necessary to check whether these patients have really understood what has been said. Providing relational care in people with limited health literacy is often even more important than in the general population. For this group of vulnerable people, the relationship with the healthcare professional is often very much in the foreground.

Many patients overestimate their level of information and understanding of health problems. This disconnect between (1) patient satisfaction with care and treatment and (2) incomplete understanding and participation in care, is greatest for (Stewart et al. 2000):

- people with limited health skills;
- people for whom speaking fluently is a problem;
- people with cognitive limitations;
- people with social disadvantages.

Nurses often encounter people with limited health skills. It is precisely these patients who often have specific patient needs. We often feel sympathy for people who are similar to us in terms of social situation and education. A telling example is that highly educated patients with an unfavorable, irregular sleeping pattern usually receive targeted attention for their problem and an adequate intervention is offered. For less educated patients and clients—the group that in fact needs it most—the intervention was limited in scope and time because the assumption was that otherwise it would not be possible for the patient to follow.

If patients or clients are in socio-economically disadvantaged situations, there are more often health inequalities and nursing support, and advocacy is more desirable for the patient and his family.

On a continuum of optimal health outcomes on the one hand versus adverse health impacts on the other hand, patients who live in unfavorable socio-economic circumstances with their families, tend to have a greater need for care.

The assessment of patient needs should be aimed at improving equity in health and at least providing appropriate care in the event of health inequality.

Nurses should identify the impact of health inequalities in assessments and intervene appropriately in order to improve quality of life and the right quality of care, with the ultimate goal of minimizing health inequalities.

10.5 Conclusion

- Vulnerable patients are a group that requires extra attention and care from healthcare professionals, especially nurses.
- Limited health literacy is a common issue among these patients, which can make it challenging for people to understand health-related information. Therefore, nurses should communicate in a way that is easily understandable and address their specific patient needs.

- Additionally, socio-economic factors can impact a patient's health outcomes, and nurses should identify and intervene appropriately to provide quality of life and minimize health inequalities.
- Overall, nurses have a crucial role in ensuring that vulnerable patients receive the care and support they need.

Box 10.1 Mind-Map Vulnerable Patients and Their Patient Needs
Create a mind-map on the importance of recognizing vulnerable patients and their specific patient needs.

Point out the difficulties vulnerable patients often face in functioning in society, also regarding less optimal health literacy.

And point out, how to pay attention to this, especially in cases of health-related decisions, to ensure effective communication and understanding.

Box 10.2 Mind-Map Socio-Economic Disadvantages on Health Outcomes
Create a mind-map on the impact of socio-economic disadvantages on health outcomes.

Point out these disadvantages and describe the relationship with (their greater need) for care.

How to identify the impact of health inequalities in assessments?

And how to intervene appropriately to provide quality of life and the right quality of care, with the ultimate goal of minimizing health inequalities?

Box 10.3 Mind-Map Identify Signs Indicating Health Disparities
Create a mind map on the importance of recognizing vulnerable patients.

Point out how to identify signs that may indicate health disparities.

Point out how you can recognize people: if I want to recognize health disparity X, then as a nurse I should be alert to …

Nursing and Person-Centered Care

11

11.1 Topic List: Patient-Centered Care

1. Definition and Importance of patient-centered care in healthcare.
2. Synonyms for patient-centered care and their significance.
3. Benefits of patient-centered care for patients and healthcare professionals.
4. Criteria for patient-centered care: respecting patient preferences, needs, and values.
5. Importance of communication in patient-centered care: Listening, understanding, and encouraging patient participation.
6. Challenges of patient-centered care: time constraints and balancing tasks in healthcare settings.
7. Impact of patient-centered care on patient satisfaction, nursing care, and well-being.
8. Elements of patient-centered care: emotional support, involving family/friends, access to healthcare, coordination, and comfort.
9. Meeting patient needs: respecting values, tailoring care, involving relatives/friends, and ensuring continuity of care.
10. Importance of understanding the patient: exploring illness experience, building patient-professional relationship.
11. Integration of patient-centered care with coordinated care: Reduction in costs, improved quality, and unified patient experiences.
12. Challenges in implementing patient-centered care: lack of consistent focus and incorporating patient characteristics/opinions.
13. Strategies for implementing patient-centered care: overcoming barriers, promoting participation, and incorporating feedback.
14. Role of healthcare professionals: developing skills, efficient delivery of patient-centered care, managing constraints.
15. Importance of patient-centered care in complex care needs: tailoring care, improving outcomes for chronic/complex conditions.

B. Sassen, *Improving Person-Centered Innovation of Nursing Care*, https://doi.org/10.1007/978-3-031-35048-1_11

11.2   Introduction

Patient-centered care is a vital aspect of modern healthcare that aims to prioritize the needs and preferences of individual patients. This approach emphasizes effective communication, collaboration, and shared decision-making between healthcare professionals and patients. By focusing on the unique needs and values of each patient, healthcare providers can improve patient satisfaction, treatment adherence, and overall health outcomes. Nurses play a crucial role in the delivery of patient-centered care, as they are often the first point of contact for patients and their families. Nurses have a unique opportunity to build strong relationships with patients and act as their advocates throughout the healthcare process. However, providing patient-centered care requires specific skills and an understanding of the patient's illness experience. Despite the benefits of patient-centered care, healthcare professionals may struggle to consistently provide it due to the complexity of the healthcare system. There can often be a mismatch between patient needs and the care provided, which can result in poor outcomes and decreased patient satisfaction. However, by assessing the extent to which the patient's perceived needs have been met and focusing on their preferences, comfort, coordination of care, emotional support, accessibility of care, information support, and family and friends, nurses can provide care that is respectful, responsive, and tailored to the individual patient's circumstances.

11.3   Outline

In this chapter, we will explore the concept of patient-centered care and how it can be achieved in practice. We will discuss the importance of effective communication and collaboration with patients, as well as the challenges and opportunities for nurses in delivering person-oriented care. By understanding the principles and practices of patient-centered care, nurses can play a critical role in improving patient outcomes and promoting high-quality healthcare. The importance of patient-centered care in nursing is a widely acknowledged concept, and it is crucial for nurses to prioritize the patient's perspective in their care. In this regard, Peplau's interpersonal relationship theory provides a framework for building a strong relationship with the patient, based on collaboration and deepening of emotional and relational ties. Patient-centered care has numerous positive impacts, such as improved patient satisfaction and self-management, and it is critical for the professional to invite the patient to participate in their care. This chapter describes the different synonyms for patient-centered care, including person-centered care, person-directed care, and person-focused care. It highlights the importance of patient-centered care in healthcare organizations, citing studies that show how patient-centered care improves patient satisfaction, quality of life, well-being, and job satisfaction for healthcare professionals. The text defines patient-centered care as an approach that respects the values, preferences, and needs of the patient, involves the patient in decision-making, and tailors care to the patient's unique circumstances. The text also discusses the challenges of providing patient-centered care, including time constraints and the complexity of the healthcare system. Finally, the text lists the prominent principles of patient-centered care, such as being holistic, respectful, aligned with the patient's dignity and values, and offering options based on the patient's right to self-determination.

11.4   Impact of Patient-/Person-Centered Care

The aim of patient-centered care is to better tailor care to the needs of the patient, also—or perhaps especially—for patients with complex care needs (Fig. 11.1). Person-centered care, patient-centered care, person-directed care, and person-focused care are all synonyms for patient-centered care.

A systematic review (Rathert et al. 2013) showed that in organizations that work more patient-centered, patients have a higher patient satisfaction with the care provided. It also turned out that patients experience a higher quality of life and a higher level of well-being. And, coupled with this, it turned out that patient-centered working also leads to more job satisfaction for healthcare professionals. The job satisfaction of care professionals is higher and the quality of care is higher (Kuipers et al. 2019).

The World Health Organization (WHO) defines patient-centered care as the Criterion Standard for Health Care. The WHO emphasizes the importance of freedom of choice and autonomy that patients have in this form of care.

The Institute of Medicine (2001) describes patient-centered care as:

Fig. 11.1 Patient-centered care. (beeldrechten: [rechten bij auteur], bestand:)

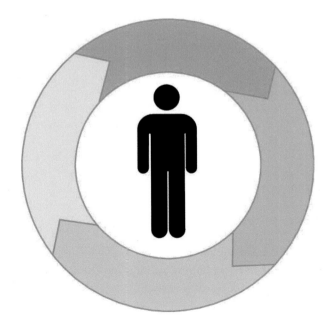

Providing care that is respectful of and responsive to individual patient preferences, needs, and values, and ensuring that this guides all clinical decisions.

Levinson et al. (2010) clearly states that professionals who applied patient-centered care paid more attention and invested more time to explore the expectations of the patient. Patient-centered professionals asked patients for their opinion, checked whether they had understood all the information and encouraged them to talk (Levinson et al. 2010). Maizes and colleagues found, however, that in time-constrained situations, patient-centered care is sacrificed in order to perform other tasks (Maizes et al. 2009).

Patient-centered care improves patient satisfaction because interaction is tailored to unique patient needs and the patient is involved in decision making. These are important elements of patient satisfaction (McCormack and McCance 2006). An RCT showed that a high degree of patient-centered working in contact moments with the patient led to a decrease in the number of contact moments. This also resulted in less specialist care, fewer hospital admissions, and fewer laboratory and diagnostic tests, and therefore also in a decrease in healthcare costs (Bertakis and Azari 2011). The most important predictor of patient satisfaction is nursing care (Laschinger et al. 2005).

Patient-centered care is about respecting the values, preferences, and needs of the patient. A vital element of patient-centered care is patient-specific health education. Patient Centered Care is about (Picker Institute IN: Davis et al. 2005):

- providing emotional support to reduce anxiety and worry;
- involving family and friends in providing care;
- access to health care;
- continuity of care with safe transitions between health care settings;
- coordinated care;
- physical comfortable care.

Patients have a number of needs that you as a nurse can meet by providing patient-centered care. First, patients need respect for their values, preferences, and stated needs. Second, they prefer coordinated and integrated care. Thirdly, they prefer support where the communication and information are specifically tailored to them. Fourth, patients need physical comfort. Fifth, patients need emotional support and need relief from anxiety and fear. Sixth, they need the involvement of their relatives and friends. And, last but not least, patients need continuity of care, even during transition (Beach et al. 2006).

Patient-centered care is an approach to care that offers the right fit with the patient's clinical needs, living conditions, and patient preferences (Rastgardani et al. 2019).

In patient-centered care, the emphasis is on understanding the patient and their unique personal circumstances; this constitutes the input for care (Baling 1968, in Morgan and Yoder 2012).

Patient- or person-centered care is a professional attitude, and it requires specific skills of the healthcare professional to make patient-centered care successful. This means to provide patient-centered care in an efficient and effective manner.

To understand a patient and provide patient-centered care in all its dimensions, you should explore the illness experience (Stewart et al. 2000). By exploring the illness experience, you come to understand the patient as a biopsychosocial, holistic entity. Only when you "know" the patient, you can work towards agreement on the care plan, including what is desirable for prevention and health promotion. The focus here is on the patient-professional relationship, where it is important to be realistic about personal and professional constraints.

When patient-centered care is combined with well-coordinated care aimed at achieving care outcomes (patient outcomes), it can lead to a reduction in costs because overuse and underuse are avoided. At the same time, the quality of care improves. When patients receive care in different settings, patient-centered care can unify patient experiences and make them less fragmented (Kuipers et al. 2019).

Patient-centered care is a care that is based on the needs and expectations of the patient and is a key element of good quality care (Bergeson and Dean 2006). However, these authors write, despite the intention and effort to improve the patient-centeredness of care and improve the quality of the professional-patient relationship, the quality of care does not automatically get better. This is because professionals do not structurally and consistently focus on the needs and concerns of their patients and clients. For example, professionals do not always bring in the characteristics and opinion of the patient as input for care and treatment. And, the treatment options are not always discussed with the patient.

An important reason for this is the complexity of the healthcare system. Because the complexity of care is increasing, patient-centered working is becoming more difficult for professionals (Bergeson and Dean 2006). Enthusiasm for patient-centered care among professionals appears to be waning over time. This means that it is getting off to a vigorous start, but over time the focus is diluting. The main factor for this is time constraints. Patients indicate that patient-centered interventions are perceived as less present over time (Rathert et al. 2013).

For patient-centered care it is (thus) about seeing the patient as a person, involving the biopsychosocial perspective in the care, making decisions together, and bearing responsibility from shared power. Starting from the relationship, entering a therapeutic alliance, forms the basis (Mead and Bower 2000). Patient-centered care is therefore a precondition for good quality care.

Peplau (1997) indicates that the interpersonal relationship is the crux of nursing, but also that this alone is not enough. The focus should be on the patient's perspective, on his illness perception, and not on the illness. The patient should be in control of his own health (Morgan and Yoder 2012), with the focus on shared partnership (Fig. 11.2).

In interpersonal nursing theory, Peplau (1997) distinguishes four successive phases in which the relationship with the patient is built: pre-interaction, orientation, collaboration (identifying the problem and exploring the problem), and completion.

Fig. 11.2 Shared partnership. (beeldrechten: [rechten bij auteur], bestand:)

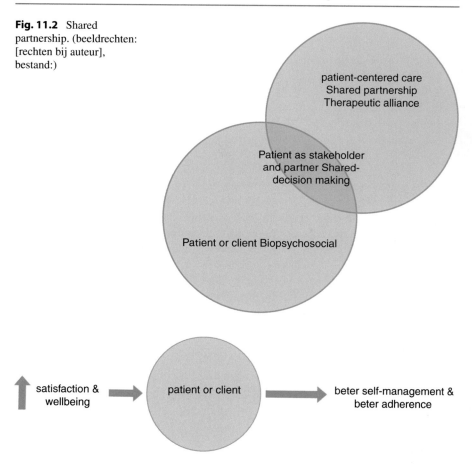

Fig. 11.3 The relationship satisfaction and well-being versus self-management and adherence. (According to: Rathert et al. 2013; beeldrechten: [rechten bij auteur], bestand:)

According to Peplau, these phases are part of a holistic relationship, where each phase leads to a deepening of the relationship with the patient, both relationally and emotionally.

A systematic literature review shows that patient-centered care has a number of positive effects (Rathert et al. 2013). It not only, as mentioned before, leads to greater patient satisfaction with care, but also—and this is very important—to better self-management of the patient. This is because the improved patient satisfaction and a better sense of well-being are the factors that lead to better adherence and better self-management and lifestyle behavior (Fig. 11.3).

Patient-centered care exists when it strengthens the patient-professional relationship, improves communication about matters that matter, helps the patient to better understand their own health, and increases patient involvement in care (Stewart et al. 2000). Good patient-centered care requires the professional to invite the patient to participate. Such an invitation could be: "I want to make sure I have helped you understand everything about your illness. What questions do you have?"

Almost all patients have questions; this is because being ill is usually complicated for them. To find out to what extent a patient has insight into their own (health) situation, you can ask: "Can you tell me what you understand? If necessary, I can then help you to explain any ambiguities." The information and advice provided should be tailored to the patient: his health, illness, and psychosocial situation (Stewart et al. 2000).

According to a literature review, patient-centered care has a number of prominent principles (Kogan et al. 2015). Person-centered care should be holistic, respectful, and aligned with the patient's dignity and values. Person-centered care should also offer the patient options, should be based on the patient's right to self-determination and should fit in with meaningful living.

To achieve this, person-centered care has a number of focus areas (McCormack et al. 2011). In a literature review, the authors mention the following points.

- First, it is about building a relationship. An important point here is to discuss the diagnosis and treatment with the patient (and his family) in such a way that trust is built up.
- Second, it is about exchanging information. Within the relationship, the patient is encouraged to ask questions. The intention is that the patient receives clear and complete information about the next steps and timing of his treatment, and that the patient is invited to provide feedback.
- Thirdly, it is about responding to emotions, such as discussing the diagnosis, because getting a diagnosis can be stressful.
- Fourth, it is about handling uncertainties, such as discussing the prognosis and the "statistics" associated with it, progress with and without treatment, and mutual coordination between professionals.
- Fifth, it is about making decisions, such as explaining why this treatment is right for this patient. The patient's preferences, such as his lifestyle and daily life, must be considered. There is cooperation to arrive at joint decision-making, whereby consideration is given to possible adverse consequences (complications) of a particular treatment. Using decision aids can provide structure and simplify the decision-making process for both patient and healthcare professional.
- Sixth, it is about the patient's self-management and lifestyle management, preparing for self-managing, aimed at optimizing health and well-being.
- Finally, it is about acknowledging that stress will elicit an emotional response in the patient. For example, in many patients the body image will change because of the disease, which can evoke anxiety and depressed feelings.

Patient-centered care has six components (Gerteis et al. 1993).

- The first component is that the healthcare professional explores the health problem of the patient and combines this with the four dimensions of the illness experience: the patient's feeling about being sick; what the patient suspects is wrong; the impact the illness has on the patient's daily life, and; patient's expectations about what should be done.

- The second component is that the healthcare professional looks at the patient as a holistic entity, with attention for biopsychosocial aspects.
- The third component is that the healthcare professional seeks agreement on what the patient wants and needs to deal with the health problem. The responsibility is not transferred to the patient, but the healthcare professional seeks agreement with the patient, tailored to the unique needs of the patient.
- The fourth component is that the healthcare professional "builds" prevention and health promotion into the patient contact.
- The fifth component is that the healthcare professional strengthens the relationship with the patient, strengthens the relationship bond and deepens contact.
- The sixth component requires that patient-centered care is realistic, so it does not raise unrealistic expectations (requires that patient-centered practice to be realistic).

Patient-centered care has a positive impact on important outcomes, such as patient satisfaction, adherence to care and treatment agreements, and self-management of chronic health problems. Patient-centered communication improves clinical outcomes in the management of diabetes, hypertension, and cancer (Levinson et al. 2010). According to patients and doctors, patient-centered care is about exchanging information, responding to emotions, dealing with uncertainties, making decisions, and enabling patients to self-manage. Patients also say that patient-centered care is about building a relationship with the doctor and that it creates a relationship in which questions about lifestyle and health risks can be asked (Gagliardi et al. 2019).

With patient-centered contact moments, the duration of the patient contact remains the same—and the time investment for the healthcare provider does not increase, contrary to what is widely believed. A big plus is that it does lead to more patient satisfaction and that the satisfaction of the healthcare professional with his work increases (Lawford et al. 2019). Another advantage is that there are fewer reports of complaints (malpractice complaints). Other benefits are that the outcomes related to the patient's health status are more favorable and that the efficiency of the care provided is assessed more positively.

Patient-centered care benefits the consultation process by clarifying the patient's concerns and needs. It also stimulates communication about treatment options and promotes empathy towards the patient (Lawford et al. 2019). Patient-centered care leads to an increase in patient satisfaction (Lawford et al. 2019). Patient-centered care also leads to a better ability of the patient to handle self-management (Lawford et al. 2019). All things considered; it, therefore, results in better health outcomes (Lawford et al. 2019).

Patient-centered care reduces length of stay and decreases readmission rates in healthcare facilities. This improves the patient's functioning and—very important— the patient experiences a better quality of life (Lor et al. 2016).

Good communication is inextricably linked to patient-centered care. This specifically requires healthcare professionals to involve the patient in the care and focus on cooperation with the patient. Patient-centered care combined with shared decision-making is at the heart of patient management in mental health care, as shown in the systematic review by Thompson and McCabe (2012).

The fact that patient-centered care is related to an improved health status of the patient is important to nurses. Associated with the improved health status, patients reported that they experienced more comfort in the relationship with the nurse, that they worried less and rated their mental well-being as more positive. The fact that patient-centered care is related to the efficiency of the care provided is important for nurses because patients had to undergo fewer diagnostic tests and fewer referrals to other healthcare professionals. The patient's perception of patient-centered contact was directly associated with these positive care outcomes (Stewart et al. 2000).

Patient- or client-centered care is based on respect for the patient as a unique person and on the moral obligation to provide care that is tailored to the person and his/her specific wishes and preferences. Patients and clients are seen as individuals with their own social world, who should be listened to, who should be correctly and fully informed, who should be respected and who should be involved in nursing care. In short, seeing the patient throughout his health care journey. This focus on individual care needs forms the starting point for good nursing care (Epstein and Street 2011).

When we look at people's lifestyles and their health behavior when they are ill, we see a diversity of patient needs and patient characteristics. However, there are no specific patient characteristics that can be predictive of whether someone is willing to collaborate with health care professionals. Patient characteristics such as age, gender, and level of education do not explain why one patient takes on his patient role in an active, participative manner, while another patient does not. Patient characteristics such as income, ethnic background and living in an urban or more rural environment also do not predict this.

What is known, is that mental health problems play a role in how people move through health care and the extent to which they are able to play an active, participatory role themselves. For example, many people with a depressive disorder or anxiety disorder have trouble with this.

Although often no clear patient characteristics can be identified, it is true that almost everyone faces difficulties when they encounter the health care system. This is all the more true if patients are required to do or refrain from doing certain things as part of the care and treatment they receive. In other words, if patients must change their lifestyle and/or health behavior (Sassen 2018a, b).

Disease-related cognitions, i.e., the perception of the disease and the view of treatment, strongly influence the way patients behave in health care. The perceived vulnerability to the disease, a disorder or limitation, plays an important role in this. In addition to this perceived vulnerability, the seriousness of the health problem also plays an important role for patients.

While for nurses the range of care and treatment for a certain patient or client group is clear and self-evident, this is usually not the case for the individual patient.

For nurses, the route that is mapped out for someone with a certain condition is self-evident; for a given health problem, the patient follows a certain route through the health care system with branches according to the type of health problem and the related impairments, limitations, and disabilities. But the route through the healthcare system can pose problems for patients. Unlike the healthcare professionals, the patient is not aware of the steps to follow and often needs a guide to stay informed about the next step in the care and treatment process. This guiding function of nurses is especially desirable because patients are not or insufficiently familiar with what to expect, which can evoke fear and unrest. Person-oriented care therefore also means that the patient experiences someone next to him, a committed nurse who is his or her guide in the health care system.

Providing patient-centered care is a continuous and dynamic process. If we look at what is desired from a patient-centered point of view, then the care should always be geared as closely as possible to the needs of the patient. Patient-centered care is care that is tailored to the moment and adapts as changes occur. There should be a match between patient needs and patient care. Is there always a good match between patient needs and patient care?

For example, if we look at the interventions aimed at promoting desired health behavior, there appears to be a regular mismatch in practice between the patient's perception (am I ill?) and the professional's intervention. Many interventions are aimed at getting the patient to work now (for example taking medicines), while this does not always correspond with the way in which the patient or client experiences or feels or needs at that moment in his disease process. There is a mismatch between the desired treatment planning and the patient's perception; there is more or less a mismatch. The nurse should constantly be aware of this perception and patient needs and use it as a starting point for nursing.

Patient-centered care can be achieved by assessing the extent to which the patient's perceived needs have been met. The nursing professional can make use of a number of main themes and questions to determine whether the care has been of sufficient quality in the following areas (Kuipers et al. 2019).

11.4.1 The Patient's Preferences

Think, among other things, of feeling that you are being taken seriously, that your wishes and preferences are being taken into account. When choosing a particular form of care and/or treatment, the patient is involved in the decision-making process. To arrive at a well-considered decision, it must be clear in advance what impact the care and treatment will have on the patient's life. Advice on this must be useful and meaningful for the patient.

11.4.2 Comfort

This point is about paying attention to pain management, fatigue, and insomnia, providing enough privacy.

11.4.3 Coordination of Care

The point here is that patients do not have to keep telling their story to the various care providers in the care and treatment process. This means that professionals ensure that they are informed and that there is coordination between professionals. On the other hand, as a patient you are aware of which healthcare professional is coordinating the care around you. The patient can contact him or her with questions. Another aspect of good coordination of care is that patient data is transferred when a referral is made, and that advices (e.g., on medication, self-management, lifestyle) is coordinated between professionals. In short, there is always and everywhere coordination in the care between professionals.

11.4.4 Emotional Support

Attention is paid to the patient's fear and anxiety and emotional support is offered. The healthcare professional considers the impact of the disease, care and treatment on (daily) life and knows the patient's needs.

11.4.5 Accessibility of Care

The patient can easily make an appointment at short notice.

11.4.6 Information Support

The patient is well informed and patient specific information is well (patient specific) explained. This includes access to your own data, such as lab results, medication overview, and referrals. And being well-informed means that as a patient you were able to ask your questions and that you received a clear answer.

11.4.7 Family and Friends

With the patient's consent, the patient's next of kin will be informed. Attention is paid to their support, and they have the opportunity to ask questions (modified Sasc questionnaire, Crohnbach's $\alpha = 0.93$; in: Kuipers et al. 2019).

Patient or client centered care is an interplay of personal, professional, and organizational relationships. Efforts to promote patient-centered care should therefore focus on the patient (and his family), on healthcare professionals and on the healthcare system (Epstein and Street 2011). In a systematic review, patient-centered care effected by fitting it within bedside rounds was not found to be ideal (Ratelle et al. 2017). This led to limited patient-centered outcomes: there was a small positive effect on patient experience and making bedside rounds had no beneficial effect on patient knowledge.

Patient-centered care provision is based on moral grounds, independent of the relationship that patient-centered care may have with health outcomes (Stewart et al. 2000).

Patient-centered communication demands certain skills from healthcare professionals. These skills have a positive impact on patient satisfaction, treatment adherence and improve self-management. From the point of view of the healthcare professional, patient-centered healthcare is defined as follows (Institute of Medicine 2001):

> […] respecting and responding to patients' wants, needs, and preferences, so they can make choices in their care that best fit their personal circumstances.

Person-centered care is care that can be characterized by continuous relationships, shared understanding, emotional support, trust, and patients who are activated and empowered to make informed decisions. Disruptions in communication are strongly associated with a greater likelihood that patients will behave differently from the recommendations associated with care and treatment. The most common patient complaints are that healthcare professionals:

- do not listen to their concerns;
- do not care about their concerns, or;
- do not provide sufficient information about their treatment (Levinson et al. 2010).

Patient-centered care starts with professionals having a greater understanding of the individual needs of the patient, their perspectives and their values. They should enable the patient to participate in care and treatment. They should build trust and mutual understanding between patient and professional (Levinson et al. 2010).

Table 11.1 provides an overview of outcomes of patient-centered care.

Table 11.1 Direct, intermediate, and health outcomes of patient-centered care

Direct outcomes	Intermediate outcomes	Health outcomes
Improved patient-centered communication during patient contact	Patient knowledge ↑	Health status ↑
	Shared-decision making ↑	Quality of life and well-being ↑
	Adherence ↑	Survival rates ↑
	Patient self-management ↑	Care disparities ↓
		Healthcare-related costs ↓

Source: Levinson et al. (2010)

Patient-centered nursing care is about making the nursing process more patient-specific by starting from patient needs. Based on the anamnesis with an exploration of the patient's needs, goals are formulated that are appropriate to the patient and his biopsychosocial circumstances. The implementation of this care plan is then measured based on the goals. The care plan in the form of a contract should be used to determine the nursing diagnosis(s) together with the patient, to jointly determine which interventions are appropriate and to evaluate them together. This evaluation takes place during the care process as well as at the end. By using the interim evaluations by building in conversation moments, the care can be adjusted to achieve and maintain optimal patient satisfaction and patient involvement.

11.5 Conclusion

- Patient-centered care is a critical aspect of high-quality healthcare that puts the patient or client unique needs and preferences at the center of care. By providing patient-centered care, healthcare professionals can improve patient satisfaction, quality of life, and overall well-being.
- Additionally, patient-centered care leads to greater job satisfaction for healthcare professionals. However, it requires specific skills and an understanding of the patient's illness experience, which can be challenging in a complex healthcare system.
- Nursing emphasizes the importance of building strong relationships with patients and clients and empowering them to take control of their own health. To build relationships with their patients, respecting their dignity and values, and aligning with meaningful living.
- Effective communication and collaboration between healthcare providers and patients are essential for achieving patient-centered care, improving patient satisfaction, adherence to treatment, and overall health outcomes. Nurses must be aware of the patient's perception of their illness and use it as a starting point for their nursing interventions, assessing the extent to which the patient's perceived needs have been met.
- Providing patient-centered care is a dynamic process that involves tailoring care to the specific needs of each patient. By focusing on the patient's preferences, comfort, coordination of care, emotional support, accessibility of care, information support, and family and friends, nursing professionals can provide care that is respectful, responsive, and tailored to the individual patient's circumstances. Ultimately, the goal of patient-centered care is to provide personalized care that respects the patient as an individual, resulting in better health outcomes and an improved quality of life.

Box 11.1 Mind-Map Patient Satisfaction and Job Satisfaction
Create a mind-map on the importance of Patient-Centered Care: point out how patient-centered care can lead to higher patient satisfaction, improved quality of life, and job satisfaction for healthcare professionals.

Box 11.2 Mind-Map Challenges Healthcare Professionals Face
Create a mind-map on challenges in providing Patient-Centered Care.
    Point out the challenges healthcare professionals face when providing patient-centered care, and look at time constraints, increasing complexity of the healthcare system, and diluting enthusiasm for patient-centered care over time. Also explore the skills and attitudes required for healthcare professionals to provide patient-centered care successfully.

Box 11.3 Mind-Map Patient-Centered Work According to the Patient
Create a mind map. Put the patient in the middle of your mind-map.
    Which themes bring about patient-centered work according to the patient. Circle the five most important themes.
    Indicate how nursing professionals can improve conditions for patient-centered care. What is the nurse supposed to do? Circle the five most important.

Nursing and Family-Centered Care

12

12.1 Topic List: The Importance of Involving Family and Friends in Patient-Centered Care

1. Patient-centered care and the role of family and friends.
2. Benefits of involving family and friends in patient care.
3. Patient and family-centered care (PFCC) and its principles.
4. Improved perceived quality of care and parent-child relationship through family-centered care.
5. Impact of communication patterns within families on patient outcomes.
6. Effects of family communication patterns on patient autonomy.
7. Culture of patient- and family-centered care and its impact on communication, patient satisfaction, safety, and quality of care.
8. Challenges and obstacles in involving family in care.
9. Key principles of negotiated care and the role of healthcare professionals in fostering mutual agreement on goals and care.

12.2 Introduction

Patient-centered care has gained significant importance in healthcare as it focuses on meeting the individual needs of patients while taking into account their social context. One crucial aspect of patient-centered care is the involvement of family and friends in the patient's or client's care. The involvement of loved ones can provide healthcare professionals with valuable insights into the patient's social context, resulting in better care that meets patient needs. This chapter highlights the importance of involving family and friends in patient care and explores the benefits of patient- and family-centered care.

12.3   Outline

This chapter discusses the importance of involving family and friends in patient-centered care. It emphasizes how involving loved ones provides healthcare professionals with valuable insight into the social context of the patient and allows them to better meet patient needs. The chapter also discusses the concept of patient and family-centered care (PFCC), which is about individualized care that respects the dignity of the patient and involves exchanging information, offering targeted patient-specific informative support, and emotional support. The benefits of PFCC are also discussed, including improved communication, better decision-making, and increased efficiency of care. The chapter also discusses the impact of communication patterns within families on patient outcomes and the importance of improving family responsiveness and support. Finally, the concept of negotiated care is introduced, which emphasizes the mutual exchange of information between the patient, family, and healthcare professional to reach mutual agreement on goals and care.

12.4   Patient- and Family-Centered Care

An important component of patient-centered care is the involvement of family and friends. Involving family and important peers provides healthcare professionals with insight into the social context of the patient. This allows care to better meet patient needs and provides reliable information about the impact of the patient's health status on the functioning of the family. Potential care needs can also be identified, for example, the overload of informal care givers, or the burden of parents of children with psychiatric health problems (Friedman 2018).

The family has an important role. In patients with Parkinson's disease, the accurate communication of *off*-symptoms is desirable to optimize the medication type and dosage and thereby improve the patient's quality of life. Patient-centered care should not only build a therapeutic relationship with the patient or client himself, but also with his family in order to get a (more) complete picture of the patient. Active listening to family members provides insight into symptoms and concerns and is an important tool for providing self-management support.

Patient- and family-centered care (PFCC) is about this patient and family involvement. It is about individualized care, which respects the dignity of the patient. It is about exchanging information, offering targeted patient-specific informative support, and offering emotional support (Gray et al. 2019).

Family-centered care improves the perceived quality of care and improves the relationship between parent and child (Lor et al. 2016). The systematic review shows that PFCC improves communication and ensures that decisions are made more deliberately. In case of contact with patients' relatives, there is a decrease in unnecessary procedures, which results in an improvement in the efficiency of care.

In a systematic review, the impact of communication patterns is described (Rosland et al. 2012). This shows that when the emphasis of communication patterns within families is on self-confidence, achievement of personal goals, family cohesion, and attentive responses to symptoms, this is associated with better patient outcomes. A positive communication pattern stimulates positive effects of care and treatment. In contrast, when the emphasis is on being critical, overprotective, controlling, and distracting responses to disease management, this was associated with negative patient outcomes. A negative communication pattern has negative effects. To improve patient outcomes, the focus should be on increasing family responsiveness and support. A positive communication pattern with relatives has a beneficial effect on the patient's autonomy.

Patient- and family-centered care as a culture within healthcare can lead to an improvement in communication and patient satisfaction, in patient safety and in the quality of care (Vermoch and Bunting 2010). However, PFCC can also provide insight into the fact that the family has a less favorable influence on the well-being of the patient, that the family does not want to be involved in the care—or at least does not want to bear responsibility—or that people in the social environment cannot bear the burden (Rastgardani et al. 2019). If the aim of your care is to work in a patient- and family-centered way, this always requires an open discussion of the possibilities to involve the family, with an eye for the obstacles that may arise for all those involved.

This is referred to as negotiated care. Negotiated care stands for the (from the start of care provision), mutual, time and time again (i.e., iterative) exchange of information between patient and his family and the professional; to reach mutual agreement on goals and care. This requires flexibility and a non-judgmental attitude from healthcare professionals (Lor et al. 2016).

12.5 Conclusion

- Patient-centered care involves the active involvement of family and friends in the patient's care. It helps healthcare professionals to understand the patient's social context, enabling them to provide better care that meets the patient's individual needs.
- Patient- and family-centered care not only improves communication and decision-making, but also leads to better patient outcomes and patient satisfaction.
- While involving family and friends in care can have numerous benefits, it is important to recognize that it may not always be feasible or desirable.
- Healthcare professionals should approach patient- and family-centered care as negotiated care, involving open discussions and mutual agreement on goals and care, and remain flexible and non-judgmental in their approach to ensure patient-centered care is maintained.

Box 12.1 Mind-Map Importance of Family and Friends in Patient-Centered Care
Create a mind-map on the Importance of Family and Friends in Patient-Centered Care.

Point out the role of family and friends in patient-centered care, benefits and side-effects.

Box 12.2 Mind-Map Communication Patterns and Patient Outcomes
Create a mind-map on communication Patterns and Patient Outcomes.

Point out the impact of communication patterns on patient outcomes. Highlight the importance of recognizing communication patterns within families and how they can affect care and treatment.

Box 12.3 Mind-Map Negotiated Care
Create a mind-map on negotiated Care.

Point out how to (mutual) exchange of information between the patient, family, and healthcare professional to reach mutual agreement on goals and care.

Emphasize how negotiated care can lead to improved patient outcomes and patient satisfaction.

Nursing and Recovery Approach

13

13.1 Topic List

1. Facilitating a Positive, Patient-Centered Relationship Based on Collaboration in the Recovery Approach.
2. Understanding the Recovery Approach: Exploring the principles and core values of the recovery approach.
3. Importance of the Therapeutic Alliance: Highlighting cooperative and collaborative relationship, including the concepts of therapeutic alliance, helping alliance, and working alliance.
4. Patient Participation and Proactive Involvement: patient participation in determining care and treatment goals, being involved in decision-making, and taking charge of behavior change and self-management for positive patient outcomes.
5. Pillars of Building an Alliance: Identifying the fundamental pillars for building a therapeutic alliance.
6. Cross-Disciplinary Cooperation: to achieve recovery-oriented care.
7. Managing Alliance Breach: strategies for strengthening the alliance and addressing breaches in the therapeutic relationship.
8. Peer and Social Support: importance of peers and important others in the patient's recovery journey,
9. Shifting from Symptom-Focused to Recovery-Focused Care.
10. Implementing Recovery-Oriented Care: Practical strategies for healthcare professionals including building a collaborative relationship, promoting patient participation, and fostering a positive therapeutic alliance.

13.2   Introduction

In mental health care, the recovery approach is aimed at facilitating a positive, patient-centered relationship based on collaboration. The focus is on recovering from previous trauma, giving meaning to the illness experience, and transcending the illness, even if it persists or recurs (Cleary et al. 2012a). The recovery approach emphasizes the patient's right to live their life on their own terms, seeking support from peers and professionals for integration into society. Building a therapeutic alliance with the patient is key to achieving this goal. This involves active participation and collaboration from both the patient and the healthcare professional. There are fundamental pillars of building an alliance. Cross-disciplinary cooperation is important, as is the role of the alliance in the recovery approach.

13.3   Outline

This chapter revolves around the importance of a positive, patient-centered relationship based on collaboration in mental health care. The recovery approach emphasizes the patient's right to live life on their own terms, seeking support from peers and professionals for integration into society. We discuss the key aspect of this approach, the importance of the therapeutic alliance between the patient and the healthcare professional, which is based on a cooperative relationship where the patient participates and is proactive in determining care and treatment goals. We discuss in this chapter the importance of building an alliance based on fundamental pillars, including empathic objectivity, focus on the present moment, respectful attention, genuine interest, and the ability to recognize conflicting goals and develop alternatives to achieve them. And also the importance of cross-disciplinary cooperation in healthcare for a recovery-oriented approach, with joint efforts aimed at patient-centered care. The alliance is working towards holistic recovery, with the emphasis on patient-centered care, with both parties encouraged to reach a consensus about treatment.

13.4   Relationship-Based Recovery

Facilitating a positive, patient-centered relationship based on collaboration is the core of the recovery approach. The patient-centered relationship in which the professional collaborates with the patient is aimed at recovery and optimizing the patient's well-being (Horsfall, et al. 2018). The recovery approach includes recovering from previous trauma, giving meaning to the illness experience and transcending the illness, even if it persists or recurs (Cleary et al. 2012a). Recovery also means the patient's right to live his life on his own terms, seeking support from peers and professionals for integration into society. The recovery approach is aimed at providing hope for the future, even if the symptoms do not go away. This approach to care is key in mental health care.

We speak of an alliance when a cooperative relationship arises between the client and the professional. We call this entering into an alliance with the patient, building a therapeutic relationship, therapeutic alliance, or helping alliance or working alliance. For a therapeutic alliance and this collaborative relationship, it is important that the patient participates and is proactive (Thompson and McCabe 2012). If the patient participates in determining the care and treatment goals, if he is involved in this decision-making and that he himself gets started with behavior change and self-management (self-manages health-behavior change), this results in positive patient outcomes (Gregory 2012).

A systematic review shows that to develop an effective alliance with the patient, it is important that there is agreement on treatment goals, there is collaborative participation and that there is regular contact between patient and professional (Thompson and McCabe 2012).

To achieve building an alliance with the patient in a shared relationship, there are a number of fundamental pillars (Arnold and Underman Boggs 2020).

- There is empathic objectivity, so that as a professional you see the patient as he is.
- There is a focus on the "here and now," on what is important to the patient at this moment and what concerns the patient has now.
- The nurse pays respectful attention, including to cultural and social differences that can influence the care treatment process.
- The nurse takes a genuine interest in the patient and communicates in a way that conveys competence and self-confidence.
- The nurse possesses the ability to recognize conflicting goals and to develop alternatives to achieve goals.

For a recovery-oriented approach, cross-disciplinary cooperation in healthcare is important, so that joint efforts are made towards the goals based on the idea of recovery (Cleary et al. 2012a, b). This is done by using a collaborative communication style of the professional and discussing the person-specific treatment and treatment elements to always get agreement from the patient (Thompson and McCabe 2012).

In the recovery approach, therefore, the core is formed by the relationship with the patient, the formation of an alliance. A breach of alliance occurs when a difference of opinion arises and there is therefore no longer agreement on the goals, when the cooperation falters or when tensions arise on an emotional level (Eubanks et al. 2018). Nurses' efforts should be directed towards strengthening the alliance (Chen et al. 2018). This can be done by starting from how the patient is feeling and examining what is going on in the therapeutic relationship at that moment (Eubanks et al. 2017).

In the alliance, the patient is not on his own but is supported by the healthcare professional and peers, important others for the patient. The alliance is working towards holistic recovery, with the emphasis on patient-centered care. Recovery means going back to functioning pre-illness.

In the past, the emphasis in mental health care was strongly on improving symptoms and on compliance with medication use, today the recovery approach is based on providing support as a professional and working together with the patient towards recovery. This may concern recovery of the functioning as it was before admission or treatment, or recovery insofar as this is possible given the impairments, limitations and/or disabilities present.

In an alliance, both parties are encouraged to reach a consensus about treatment. This by communicating patient-oriented, which does justice to the preferences of the patient. Alliance is about the patient-professional relationship and the mutual interaction that takes place in this relationship, the mutual bond that arises, the goals, the treatment plan, and the agreements.

13.5 Conclusion

- The recovery approach in mental health care is centered on building a positive, patient-centered relationship based on collaboration. The formation of a therapeutic alliance between the patient and healthcare professional is critical to achieving this goal.
- A strong alliance is based on empathic objectivity, respectful attention, genuine interest, and the ability to recognize conflicting goals and develop alternatives to achieve them.
- Cross-disciplinary cooperation is important to ensure joint efforts towards the patient's recovery goals.
- In an alliance, both parties work together to reach a consensus about treatment, with a focus on patient-oriented communication and the preferences of the patient.
- A strong alliance is key to facilitating recovery and optimizing the patient's well-being.

Box 13.1 Mind-Map Collaborative Relationship Building
Create a mind-map on the importance of patient-centered care and collaborative relationship building in mental health care.

Point out the importance of a positive, patient-centered relationship based on collaboration between the patient and the healthcare professional. Use: recovery and optimization of the patient's well-being vs. symptom improvement and medication compliance, shared decision-making, empathy, and mutual respect.

Box 13.2 Mind-Map On Key Pillars of Therapeutic Alliance
Create a mind-map on key pillars of therapeutic alliance.
Point out the pillars that should be the foundation of the therapeutic alliance,
Point out how nurses should handle these pillars.

Box 13.3 Mind-Map Maintaining and Strengthening the Alliance
Create a mind-map on strategies for maintaining and strengthening the alliance.
Point out strategies that can help maintain and strengthen the alliance.
Take into account cross-disciplinary cooperation in healthcare, as well as the role of peers and important others in the recovery process.

Box 13.4 Mind-Map Recovery-Oriented Professional Practice
Create a mind map. Put the similarities and differences of patient-centered professional practice (left) and recovery-oriented professional practice (right). Circle the three similarities that are most important to you.

Nursing and Co-Creation of Care

14

14.1 Topic List for Co-Creation of Care Can Improve Care Outcomes

1. Importance of co-creation of care for patients with complex care needs, such as multimorbidity.
2. Co-creation of care as a strategy for addressing uncertainty in care outcomes.
3. How co-creation of care can improve patient satisfaction and well-being; improving health outcomes and care results.
4. Building and maintaining the relationship in co-creation of care: agreement on goals, shared knowledge, and mutual respect.
5. Co-creation of care as a means of searching for innovative solutions for complex problems.
6. Overcoming challenges and barriers to implementing co-creation of care in healthcare settings.
7. Importance of incorporating co-creation of care as a standard practice in healthcare settings to improve overall care quality.
8. The role of technology and digital health in facilitating co-creation of care.
9. Future directions for co-creation of care in healthcare settings.

14.2 Introduction

In healthcare, patient-centered care has always been an essential aspect of delivering effective and quality care. However, with the increasing complexity of healthcare needs and the rise of patients with multimorbidity, healthcare professionals are now turning towards co-creation of care to improve patient outcomes. Co-creation of care is a collaborative approach to healthcare where the healthcare provider and the patient work together to build a relationship that is centered around the patients' or clients' unique needs, goals, and preferences. This approach is particularly crucial when uncertainty surrounds the care process or when caring for patients with complex care needs. Co-creation of care has clear benefits and can lead to improved patient outcomes.

14.3   Outline

This chapter discusses the concept of co-creation of care in healthcare and its importance for improving care outcomes, especially for patients with complex care needs such as those with multimorbidity. It explains that co-creation of care is about building a relationship between the healthcare professional and the patient in which there is patient-centered interaction and communication, focusing on the individual, unique patient. The chapter highlights that co-creation of care leads to higher patient satisfaction with care, greater patient well-being, and better health outcomes, as it optimizes the quality of patient-centered interaction and communication. Additionally, it emphasizes the importance of building and maintaining the relationship, agreement on goals, shared knowledge, and mutual respect for each other's points of view. However, it notes that co-creation of care requires an investment of time from the healthcare professional, especially for patients with multimorbidity, who may need more attention and care due to the complexity of their health conditions.

14.4   Patient's Role in Co-Creation

In addition to patient-centered care, co-creation of care can improve care outcomes.

- Co-creation of care is especially important for complex care and complex care needs of the patient. Think of people with multimorbidity who are having multiple health problems at the same time, where care and treatment for one health problem is sometimes not in line with the care and treatment of another health problem.
- Co-creation of care is also an obvious choice if there is uncertainty as to whether the type of care provided will lead to the desired result.
- Co-creation of care can also be used if there is uncertainty as to whether the care will properly meet the needs and wishes of the patient (Kuipers et al. 2019).

Co-creation of care is a way of communicating in situations of uncertainty about the effects of care and treatment, and when there are limitations in time (Kuipers et al. 2019).

Co-creation relates to complex issues, such as loneliness among people with psychiatric health problems, or increasing the care independence of people with chronic diseases.

Co-creation of care leads to higher patient satisfaction with care as well as to greater patient well-being, and specifically to higher social well-being. Co-creation of care leads to better health outcomes, and it leads to better care results. These effects arise because the quality of patient-centered interaction and communication is optimized by the healthcare professional (Kuipers et al. 2019).

For the co-creation of care, the relationship between the professional and the patient plays an important role. Co-creation of care is about building a relationship with the patient in which there is patient-centered interaction and communication. In doing so, the healthcare professional focuses on the individual, unique patient. If this positive interaction and communication arises, there is a co-creation of care and patient-centered working together (Kuipers et al 2019).

Within the co-creation of care, care remains goal-oriented and therefore productive. Productive, purposeful patient-centered interaction is communication that is timely, frequent, accurate, and problem-solving (Kuipers et al. 2019).

In addition to the emphasis on interaction and communication, co-creation of care is about building and maintaining the relationship: agreement on goals, shared knowledge, and mutual respect for each other's points of view. This means that the patient influences the care process and its results.

Together, healthcare professionals and patients search for innovative solutions for complex problems.

Co-creation of care always requires an investment of time from the healthcare professional, for example, in the case of people with multimorbidity. This is because the health care system is less well geared to this patient group, with the result that there is a higher risk of undesirable effects when treating people with multiple health problems (Kuipers et al. 2019).

14.5 Conclusion

- Co-creation of care is an effective way to improve patient outcomes, especially for those with complex care needs.
- This collaborative approach fosters a positive and productive relationship between the healthcare provider and the patient, where the patient's unique needs, goals, and preferences are taken into consideration.
- As a result, the quality of patient-centered interaction and communication is optimized, leading to better health outcomes, patient satisfaction, and social well-being.
- While co-creation of care requires an investment of time from healthcare professionals, it is a worthwhile investment that can lead to better healthcare outcomes for patients with complex care needs.
- It is essential for healthcare professionals to adopt a co-creation of care approach to ensure the best possible care for their patients.

Box 14.1 Mind-Map Benefits of Co-Creation of Care
Create a mind-map on key benefits of co-creation of care for patients with complex care needs.

Point out main problems of people having complex needs.

Point out the benefits of co-creation of care, and how this may lead to better health outcomes and higher patient satisfaction.

Box 14.2 Mind-Map Challenges Co-Creation of Care
Create a mind-map on challenges faced by healthcare professionals in implementing co-creation of care, particularly in the case of patients with multimorbidity.

How can these challenges be addressed (to ensure that patients receive the best possible care?)

Box 14.3 Mind-Map Relationship-Building in Co-Creation of Care
Create a mind-map on communication and relationship-building in co-creation of care.

Point out how healthcare professionals can ensure that they are communicating effectively with their patients and building positive, productive relationships that lead to better care outcomes?

Box 14.4 Mind-Map Similarities and Differences Person-Centered Care and Co-Creation of Care
Make a mind map of the similarities and differences between person-centered care and co-creation of care.

Point out what is 'added' to person-centered care, when applying co-creation of care.

And what does this "extra" ask given the professional attitude of the nurse professional?

Nursing and Autonomy and Self-Direction

15

15.1 Topic-List: Importance of Autonomy in Care

1. Caregiving Paradigm Shift towards Patient Autonomy.
2. Understanding the Paradigm Shift in Caregiving: From Paternalism to Autonomy.
3. Autonomy as a Key Element in Patient-Centered Care.
4. Patient Autonomy and its Importance in Caregiving, Balancing Patient Needs and Preferences, Reducing Patient Vulnerability, Empowerment and Enhancing Patient Decision-Making.
5. Culturally Competent Care and Autonomy.
6. Autonomy in Caregiving: Challenges and Strategies for Healthcare Professionals.
7. Relational care and its importance in nursing practice, Autonomy as a key aspect of relational care.
8. Moral distress as a common ethical issue faced by nursing professionals Inner and outer restrictions that can cause moral distress and affect autonomy in nursing.
9. External factors that can contribute to moral distress in nursing, such as technology, staffing, communication, leadership pressure, and patient demands.
10. Goals of improving moral competences of nursing professionals, including handling moral problems, explicit reasoning, interprofessional dialogue, and improving management.
11. Ethical problems arising from conflicts between perceived best actions and inability to carry them out in practice.
12. Factors contributing to moral distress in nursing, such as high workload, improper drug dispensing, poor communication, lack of support from

organization, failure to respect patients' rights and autonomy, and dealing with death and complicated communication with families.

13. Moral deliberation or moral case deliberation as a strategy for addressing moral dilemmas in nursing practice for finding solutions to moral problems.

15.2   Introduction

The way caregivers provide care to patients has evolved over time from a paternalistic, disease-oriented approach to a patient-centered approach, focusing on patient autonomy, preferences, cultural values, and needs. Autonomy involves patients making their own decisions, in consultation with healthcare professionals and family. The patient's autonomy and self-confidence reduce their vulnerability and increase their ability to participate in their care, which can improve their quality of life. Caregivers need to adopt a person-centered, patient-centered, family-centered, and culturally competent care model to support the patient's coping skills and decision-making abilities.

The provision of healthcare should not be viewed as the sole responsibility of healthcare professionals, but rather a collaborative effort between the healthcare provider and the patient. The clinical relationship between the two parties should be built on empathy and trust rather than a paternalistic attitude. This approach enables patients to have a say in the decision-making process and to feel autonomous, which is especially important for patients who have lost control due to illness or hospitalization.

Patients should have as much control as possible over their own health, which can be achieved through self-direction and self-management. Nurses play a significant role in providing relational care and advocacy for patients. However, ethical issues may arise, causing moral distress for nurses. Despite the challenges, it is important for nurses to stand up for the patient's interests and be an integral part of healthcare provision. Overall, a patient-centered approach is crucial to creating positive healthcare outcomes.

15.3   Outline

This chapter discusses the paradigm shift in caregiving from a paternalistic, disease-oriented perspective to a patient-focused approach that emphasizes patient autonomy, patient needs, preferences, and cultural values. The importance of autonomy, self-regulation, and patient empowerment is highlighted in the text. The role of nurses in caregiving is discussed, emphasizing the need for a person-centered, patient-centered, family-centered, and culturally competent care model. The importance of collaborative relationships between healthcare professionals and patients, the impact of patient satisfaction on quality of life, and the need for healthcare organizations to view professionals as the means to treat patients and clients are also discussed. The text suggests that empowering patients with knowledge, skills, and self-awareness to take control of their own lives can lead to better health outcomes and higher patient satisfaction.

15.4 Autonomy of Patients and Clients

Caregiving has shown a paradigm shift from a paternalistic, disease-oriented perspective to a model of care with a focus on patient autonomy, patient needs, preferences, and cultural values.

Paternalism refers to the dominant role of professionals who determine what is best for the patient. Autonomy means that the patient himself—in or after consultation with professionals and possibly family—determines what is best for himself (Abdei-Tawab and Roter 2002).

Welford et al. (2012) expresses this contradiction as follows:

Patients' autonomy is threatened by professional paternalism and institutional self-interest.

Autonomy is about freedom, independence, self-determination, and self-government (Welford et al. 2012). Autonomy can also be seen as a capacity to be able and to dare to make decisions. Autonomous decision-making then forms the core (Welford et al. 2012). The capacity to make decisions is decision-specific, which means that patients may not be able to act completely autonomously but can always opt for specific (partial) decisions.

Autonomy also stands for independence, acting in accordance with one's own morality, as opposed to acting under the influence of others.

Along with self-confidence, autonomy reduces patients' vulnerability. Both skills enhance patients' ability to participate in care and make decisions. By participating, patients can provide input to care and perform patient management previously done by professionals (Suhonen et al. 2000), thereby also developing their self-management.

Empowerment can increase a patient's autonomy and self-confidence. This may involve mastering strategies to acquire information, strategies to support individual choices, strategies to communicate effectively and to be able to negotiate. Patients who have this knowledge feel equipped to make health-related decisions (Morgan and Yoder 2012).

Autonomy in care is at the heart of care where the self-esteem of the patient is honored, regardless of their physical or psychosocial circumstances. Autonomy leads to patient satisfaction in patients:

- if the patient's autonomy is properly considered, the patient experiences a high degree of satisfaction with the care. This high patient satisfaction in turn increases the experienced quality of life.
- if patients' autonomy is limited, which is more often the case when a lot of routine care is provided, patient satisfaction with care decreases. This limited autonomy leads to reduced patient satisfaction and has a negative impact on quality of life (Welford et al. 2012).

Professionals should focus on the autonomy of the patient and allow their way of providing care to be guided by autonomy, dignity and personhood. And in patients for whom or in situations in which autonomy is not or not entirely possible, they should constantly seek the balance to what can be an autonomous decision by the patient. For example, care providers can offer people with a high degree of care dependence, options regarding daily life and daily care, and; not just providing routine care (Welford et al. 2012).

According to Illich, the medical profession is an emphatically present profession within the health care sector. The medical profession tends to exercise power (professional power) and thus make patients dependent (dependency cultures) by detaching them from their own problem-solving abilities (disabling). The professional has the authority to determine the problem. The human being is transformed into a patient who must be saved by the expert. According to Illich, this creates an undesirable situation in which the human being (the patient or client) can do little or nothing and is at the mercy of the healthcare professional and the healthcare system. To get out of this undesirable situation, Illich advocates a post-professional ethos, in which the patient must be held accountable for his own self-reliance.

From the perspective of self-regulation, each patient responds with a targeted response (coping response) to (the threat posed by) illness. The patient experiences a health threat and wants to counter this threat with an adequate response through self-regulation.

What that coping response looks like is up to the patient to decide for himself. Everyone can and will choose their own way to deal with the threat to health. The self-regulatory perspective broadly influences how the patient deals with illness and health. It requires a coping response from the patient when he receives a referral: he determines whether or not there is a health problem in his opinion. Another coping response occurs after hearing an unfavorable diagnosis. Dealing with recommendations regarding care and treatment also requires a coping response from patients: do I act on these recommendations, to a certain extent or not at all? Am I able to put the recommendations into practice, and if so, how can I best do that?

From this perspective, nursing professionals focus on the patient's coping skills. These skills indicate what is desirable in a broad sense to deal with the disease: all kinds of thoughts, ideas, and skills.

Nursing professionals must change their orientation: not a paternalistic, patronizing perspective, but act according to a person-centered, patient-centered, family-centered, and culturally competent care model (Lor et al. 2016). Culturally competent care is care that is tailored to a specific patient population. In all these care models, the aim is to establish collaborative relationships. These relationships consist of individual healthcare professionals and inter-professional healthcare teams who collaborate with the patient and their family in the planning and implementation of care (Lor et al. 2016). Collaborative relationships are forged by providing honest information about the patient and about the care (Lor et al. 2016).

Patient empowerment can be seen as taking control of one's own life. Patients become empowered (morally stronger) if they have the knowledge, skills, and a certain degree of self-awareness to influence their own behavior and improve their quality of life. Patients who feel empowered, experience higher patient satisfaction with care, higher adherence, and better health outcomes.

Empowerment can be created by entering a relationship with the patient and by showing an open attitude, personal interest, and understanding for the other person. It is all about equality and mutual respect. Patient and professional take the time to sit together to understand the other; one has the will to be there for the other. It is about the willingness to help the other person. And, research shows that people having a depression rated their care as more effective if the healthcare professional developed a close relationship with them (Fig. 15.1) (Morgan and Yoder 2012).

Healthcare organizations should not see professionals as the provider of care, but as the means to treat patients and clients. The relationship offers important opportunities for creating positive outcomes in healthcare. By entering and deepening the relationship with the patient, it can become clear what goals the patient sets in his life. Through conversation, patients can become aware of their ambivalent attitudes in treatment and explore positive and negative issues associated with treatment. The clinical relationship should be built on empathy and trust. This contrasts with a paternalistic attitude. Patients should feel free to ask questions to shape their own opinion and be autonomous.

For nursing professionals, an important perspective on care is that patients take control of their own health as much as possible. This starts with nurses focusing on ensuring that a patient loses control as little as possible. And with patients who have lost (part of) control, they focus on restoring this control. For example, in people with psychiatric health problems, it is about recovery and regaining control.

The provision of care should be aimed at ensuring that patients maintain firm control over themselves. And if their hands become loose (or loosened) from this control, nurses do everything they can to ensure that these patients tighten their grip (again) and take control of their own health within their capabilities.

Why is this so important? When a patient loses control of his life, he finds himself in a situation which is referred to as hospitalization. You speak of hospitalization when a person who has been admitted to a healthcare facility adapts to the rules and habits that apply in this facility. Someone goes to the hospital for hip surgery, puts on his pajamas and goes to bed; after all, he is a patient.

This also appears to happen with people who are admitted to a nursing home or a psychiatric hospital. With such an admission, people feel that they are "immersed" in the structure of the healthcare institution. People let go of their own control and often because of the unfamiliarity with "how things are done" they adopt a wait-and-see attitude. They feel overwhelmed, which sets in motion a process in which

Fig. 15.1 Paternalism versus autonomy of the patient. (beeldrechten: [rechten bij auteur] bestand:)

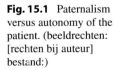 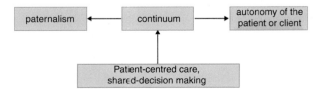

self-direction is no longer paramount. A pattern of adaptation to the situation in which people find themselves emerges.

Naturally, every social situation with others requires adjustments: people in a family, at work, also adapt. The difference is that the patient tends to relinquish control too much, becomes increasingly accustomed to the health care system and gets hospitalized.

Patient-centered care is strongly linked to patient autonomy and seeing the patient as autonomous regarding decision making (Gill et al. 2019). According to the deliberative model, deliberation and negotiation can promote the patient's autonomy. Think of discussing new ideas or insights. The patient and professional are jointly responsible for discussing the consequences of a decision, including the advantages and disadvantages and the possible use of (health care) facilities.

Patient-centered care is also about involving family in the care. Particularly with children, input from family can be of great value in determining the child's preferences. Sometimes, however, the child's preferences are different from the parents. According to the deliberative model, the child should be the point of departure for care. The degree to which the child plays a role in the decision-making process depends on age, competence, and care needs.

Patients should therefore have as much as possible control over living with a (chronic) health problem. The current structure of healthcare makes this increasingly easy, but also more and more necessary. This is because care and treatment are increasingly being offered without or with as short a stay as possible in (psychiatric) hospitals. Care is increasingly ambulatory, the patient stays at home and, if necessary, goes to a general practitioner, an outpatient clinic or a short-term hospitalization setting. Most of the time, therefore, the patient is at home, managing his health at home and dealing with his illness in the context of daily life. In this home context, the patient will monitor his health himself, will live his life with his health problem and will do the things that have a favorable influence on his health situation. Self-direction then translates into dealing with daily life in such a way that your illness affects you as little as possible. Self-management then occupies a crucial place in self-direction or restoring one's own direction.

Baart (2018) states that providing relational care is only possible if the care recipient has a continuous and direct influence on the care. The patient must be able to indicate his wishes and needs at any time: "this is what I want, and this is not"; this is good for me and that is not good for me; "this suits my lifestyle and that is not me" and so on. Providing relational care means that the care receiver has a say in and influence in the relationship with the nurse.

Regarding autonomy, but also for a large number of other matters, nursing professionals can experience moral distress. These are ethical issues that pose a threat to the integrity of nurses and to the quality of care. Barlem and Ramos (2014) put it this way:

What the nurse thinks is the right thing to do and some (inner or outer) restriction.

Characteristic here is that situations that evoke personal moral distress (inner moral distress) affect the nurse's autonomy and/or make it difficult or even impossible for him or her to stand up for the patient's interests as an integral part of the nursing care. This standing up for the patient's interests (patient advocacy) is an important aspect of healthcare provision.

When defending the patient's interests, nursing professionals may encounter obstacles, both from the organization and from hierarchical relationships. But instead of asking why distress is experienced, it is better to ask yourself why you would accept certain situations as immutable or 'just part of the game" (Barlem and Ramos 2014).

Matters that evoke external moral distress include the impact of technology, lack of staff, lack of communication, leadership pressure, too many patients, excessive (impossible) requirements, and the increasing demand from patients or the pressure to provide good quality care. This can occur when treating a terminally ill patient, when unnecessary examinations are carried out, when colleagues treat people inadequately, when there is a power relationship between professionals and when there is a lack of support for professionals from within the organization.

It is not easy to do justice to the autonomy of the patient. It is also not easy to properly integrate patient-centered care and shared decision-making into care, due to the high ethical demands placed on professionals in this regard (Gill et al. 2019).

The moral dilemma arises from clinical practice and revolves around the question:

"What is the morally right thing to do and how do we do it correctly?"

Improving the moral competences of professionals aims to improve the quality of to improve care. But this is not the only thing. Other goals are (Molewijk et al. 2008; Weidema et al. 2012):

– the ability to handle moral problems;
– making explicit the motives of professionals for doing something in a certain way;
– creating a culture in which professionals enter into a dialogue with each other (also with colleagues from other disciplines);
– increasing the quality of management.

Ethical problems arise when professionals perceive something as a problem or conflict, but they are unable to make a choice as to what they can do best in the case in question. Such cases make the job unpleasant. There is a dilemma: a situation has arisen in which it is impossible to carry out the ethically adequate action (Barlem and Ramos 2014). The nurse, therefore, knows what is right to do but is unable to do so due to obstacles such as a lack of time, unwilling managers or colleagues, a hierarchical structure that makes action impossible, bureaucratic obstacles or a lack of agreement between colleagues (Barlem and Ramos 2014).

Moral distress is related to (Barlem and Ramos 2014):

– high workload and non-optimal personnel management;
– improper drug dispensing (not or too much);
– interpersonal relationships at work with whom there is poor or no communication;
– lack of support from the organization for nurse autonomy;
– failure to respect patients' rights;

- failure to respect patients' autonomy;
- death is a source of stress, especially when related to professional inadequate care and associated complicated communication with the family;
- providing unnecessary care.

Moral deliberation or moral case deliberation is the collective discussion of perspectives on a moral problem with professionals. A systematic reflection takes place by professionals on a moral dilemma. This moral problem (dilemma) is often "wrapped up" in a case description (Weidema et al. 2012). During moral deliberation, the perspectives of others are related to one's own (individual) perspective and a solution is sought in this way (Barlem and Ramos 2014).

15.5 Conclusion

- The paradigm of caregiving has shifted from a paternalistic, disease-oriented perspective to a person-centered, patient-centered, family-centered, and culturally competent care model. This model aims to establish collaborative relationships with individual healthcare professionals and inter-professional healthcare teams who work with the patient and their family in the planning and implementation of care.
- Autonomy, self-confidence, and empowerment are central concepts in this model. Care providers should focus on the autonomy of the patient, allow their way of providing care to be guided by autonomy, dignity, and personhood, and constantly seek the balance between what can be an autonomous decision by the patient.
- Patient empowerment can be achieved through knowledge, skills, and a supportive environment that provides patients with choices and options.
- Providing relational care to patients in healthcare and the role of healthcare professionals in advocating for their patients can improve autonomy and empowerment.
- Moral distress that healthcare professionals can experience when faced with ethical issues that affect the quality of care can threaten their autonomy.
- Moral deliberation can improve moral competences of healthcare professionals to handle moral problems, this improve the quality of care, and create a culture of dialogue among healthcare professionals.
- Factors that can cause moral distress among healthcare professionals are high workload, improper drug dispensing, poor interpersonal relationships, lack of support from the organization, failure to respect patients' rights and autonomy, and providing unnecessary care.
- This emphasizes the importance of ethical considerations in healthcare and the need for healthcare professionals to have the skills and knowledge to navigate moral dilemmas.

Box 15.1 Mind-Map The Paradigm Shift
Create a mind-map on the paradigm shift in caregiving.

Point out how the caregiving approach has shifted from a paternalistic, disease-oriented perspective to a model of care that focuses on patient autonomy, needs, preferences, and cultural values. Use: advantages and challenges of this shift in terms of patient satisfaction, quality of care, and outcomes.

Box 15.2 Mind-Map Autonomy in Caregiving
Create a mind-map on autonomy in caregiving.

Point out the importance of patient participation in decision-making.

Point out the role of healthcare professionals in supporting autonomy.

Use: how patients' self-confidence and autonomy can be enhanced, and the impact of limited autonomy on patient satisfaction.

Box 15.3 Mind-Map Empowerment and the Healthcare Relationship
Create a mind-map on patient empowerment and the healthcare relationship.

Point out how patient empowerment can lead to improved patient satisfaction, adherence, and health outcomes, and the importance of a deepening relationship between the patient and the healthcare professional in achieving these outcomes.

Box 15.4 Mind-Map Autonomy and Self-Direction
Make a mind map and focus on autonomy and self-direction.

Which factors have a positive influence (place it on the left) and which factors have a negative influence (place it on the right)? Which factors are most important to you personally?

Box 15.5 Mind-Map Inner and Outer Moral distress Eliciting Factors
Create a mind map on inner and outer moral distress eliciting factors.

Place the inner moral distress eliciting factors on top of the top hemisphere of your mind map. Place the outer moral distress triggers in the lower hemisphere of your mind map.

Do not limit yourself to general health care, but also include mental health care.

For each factor, place a solution to deal with the inner and outer moral distress.

Nursing and Shared Decision-Making 16

16.1 Topic List: Shared Decision-Making in Healthcare

1. Exploring shared decision-making and its importance in patient care.
2. Patient Preferences and Involvement: Preference of patients for shared or autonomous decision-making.
3. Challenges in Shared Decision-Making.
4. Steps in Shared Decision-Making: Outlining the sub-steps involved in shared decision-making.
5. Role of Decision Aids: Supporting shared decision-making, particularly in providing risk calculations and individual feedback to help patients make informed choices.
6. Mental Health Care and Shared Decision-Making: Unique challenges and benefits.
7. Impact on Patient Quality of Life.
8. Building a collaborative relationship based on mutual trust between healthcare professionals and patients in shared decision-making.
9. Barriers to Shared Decision-Making: Identifying barriers to implementing shared decision-making, and discussing strategies to overcome them.
10. Future Directions and implications of shared decision-making in healthcare.

16.2 Introduction

Shared decision-making has emerged as an important approach in healthcare to involve patients in their care process and treatment decisions. The focus is on creating a collaborative relationship between healthcare professionals and patients that respects the patient's preferences and values. The aim is to provide individualized care that takes into account the patient's unique needs and circumstances. Shared decision-making is particularly relevant in serious illness situations where quick decisions need to be made. This approach can be facilitated by decision aids and tools that support patient involvement and understanding.

16.3   Outline

This chapter discusses shared decision-making in healthcare, which involves offering treatment options and investigations to the patient and allowing them to choose what they want. It emphasizes that shared decision-making is more than just making treatment choices, but it should be integrated throughout the care process to tailor treatment to the patient's preferences and improve their perceived quality of life. The involvement of both the patient and the healthcare professional is essential for shared decision-making, and it requires a collaborative relationship based on mutual trust. The passage also discusses the challenges that arise when decisions have to be made quickly, especially in the case of serious illnesses. Decision aids can support decision-making by providing patients with risk calculations and individual feedback, and they encourage patient involvement. Finally, the chapter notes that shared decision-making is also important in mental health care.

16.4   Patient's Part in Shared Decision-Making

Shared decision-making may involve offering possible treatments or investigations, whereby the patient can choose what he wants. But shared decision-making is more than making well-considered treatment choices: it is important throughout the care process and should be integrated into patient care. This is because making joint decisions about care and treatment, specifically tailored to the preferences of the patient, has an important influence on the perceived quality of life of patients and clients. Consider, for example, incorporating patient preferences into the chemotherapy treatment schedule, so that "good days" are spared for important moments within the family or at work (Chewning et al. 2012).

Involvement of both the patient and the professional is indispensable for shared decision-making. The majority of patients prefer shared or autonomous decision-making. There is only a very small group of patients who delegate decisions. This concerns patients who are unable to participate in decisions or do not want to (at that time). If patient involvement does not arise, this may be the result of the professional's lack of skills to involve the patient in the decision-making process, or of a lack of time, or the experience of a lack of time on the part of the professional (Chewning et al. 2012; Sassen 2023).

Shared decision-making is about entering into a relationship, an alliance between healthcare professional and the patient or client. At its core, this collaborative relationship revolves around mutual trust that must be felt by the patient (Sassen 2023). The greatest challenge for shared decision-making arises when the patient is confronted with a serious illness and decisions have to be made quickly (Maizes et al. 2009).

Shared decision-making can be simplified by going through a number of substeps. We start with inviting the patient to give his opinion in the conversation and to indicate that the patient has been invited to make a choice. The exploration consists of the healthcare professional ensuring a joint understanding of the disease. The healthcare professional then presents the treatment options. The healthcare professional explores the patient's needs and explores lifestyle factors. After this, the healthcare professional presents the treatment options, invites you to exchange thoughts, and makes a choice (Chewning et al. 2012).

Decision aids can support decision-making, especially if linked to risk calculations. For example, if a patient learns that his risk of mortality is reduced by 7% with a particular intervention, he can decide whether this risk reduction is worth starting a therapy. If a decision aid maps out the risk reduction and provides the patient with individual feedback, he or she can make an informed decision on this basis (Maizes et al. 2009). Decision support tools also encourage patient involvement (Thompson and McCabe 2012).

In mental health care, the nature of the symptoms makes it more difficult to make shared decisions. Nevertheless, this branch of healthcare also strives for collaborative communication, both during consultation and throughout the treatment process. A systematic review shows that shared decision-making is a useful communication model to improve patient involvement in the decision-making processes within consultations in mental health care, although this does not always lead to adherence directly.

16.5 Conclusion

- Shared decision-making is a fundamental approach in healthcare that aims to involve people in their care process and treatment decisions.
- It is about creating a collaborative relationship between healthcare professionals and patients that respects the patient's preferences and values.
- Patients who are involved in the decision-making process have better outcomes and a better quality of life.
- Decision aids and tools that support patient involvement and understanding can facilitate shared decision-making.
- Mental health care is also recognizing the importance of shared decision-making in improving patient involvement in decision-making processes.
- Moving forward, healthcare organizations should prioritize training and resources to support shared decision-making and ensure that patients receive the highest quality care possible.

Box 16.1 Mind-Map Shared Decision-Making in Patient Care
Create a mind-map about the importance of shared decision-making in patient care.

Point out the importance of shared decision-making throughout the care process and how it can improve the perceived quality of life of patients and clients.

And, point out the benefits of incorporating patient preferences into treatment schedules, especially in cases of serious illnesses.

Box 16.2 Mind-Map Patient Involvement in Decision-Making
Create a mind-map on factors that influence patient involvement in decision-making.

Point out reasons why patient involvement in decision-making might not occur. Explore factors such as the professional's (lack of) skills or time, as well as patient preferences.

Box 16.3 Mind-Map Strategies to Support Shared Decision-Making
Create a mind-map on strategies and tools to support shared decision-making.

Point out the different sub-steps involved in shared decision-making.

Indicate how to use decision aids in supporting decision-making and encouraging patient involvement, also applicable for mental health care.

Nursing and Self-Management

17

17.1　Topic List

1. Importance of patient compliance in healthcare.
2. Burden of chronic health problems and adherence to treatment plans.
3. Patient outcomes and the influence of treatment compliance.
4. Self-management and symptom management in chronic health conditions.
5. Challenges in self-management and the role of nurses in supporting patients.
6. Disease management and self-management support.
7. Definition of self-management and its significance for nurses.
8. Challenges in current healthcare system and health promotion.
9. Multimorbidity and impact on self-management and treatment adherence.
10. Patient perspective on following recommendations and information provision.
11. Factors influencing patient adherence and the biomedical model of health.
12. Solutions for improving patient self-management and communication.
13. Benefits of patient-centered care and person-centered communication.
14. Strategies for integrating health promotion and prevention in nursing care.

17.2　Introduction

Patient-centered care is an approach to healthcare that involves adopting an individualized and holistic biopsychosocial approach to patient management. It requires healthcare professionals to offer physical and psychosocial support and communicate in a way that empowers patients, thereby stimulating patient management. This approach also includes self-management, which involves helping patients adopt new or change existing behaviors to improve their health. Adherence to treatment in mental health care is twice as high if professionals are good communicators, and medication-specific discussions may improve adherence. Patient self-management affects prognosis, and healthcare professionals must work toward optimal health outcomes. The extent to which patients comply with the recommended treatment plan plays a significant role in achieving the desired patient outcomes.

The concept of disease management has become increasingly important in healthcare, with the focus on supporting patients in self-care and self-management throughout the entire care pathway. This involves disease prevention, early detection, symptom reduction, prevention of worsening symptoms, promotion of optimal self-management, and encouraging a healthy lifestyle. Self-management support and promotion require customization and a commitment to health promotion and prevention from healthcare professionals, particularly nurses. However, patients' ability to adopt the advice and recommendations provided by healthcare professionals can be challenging, especially for those with multiple health problems. Communication between healthcare professionals and patients must be person-centered to promote patient self-management successfully. Despite the increasing number of people with chronic diseases, health promotion and prevention receive little attention and budget in the healthcare sector. If the focus shifts to supporting patients' balance in maintaining health and promoting and optimizing their quality of life and life expectancy, the principles of disease prevention and health promotion could be better applied in nursing care.

17.3 Outline

This chapter revolves around patient-centered care and its relationship with adherence to treatment. Patient-centered care involves an individualized and holistic approach to patient management by healthcare professionals, using a communication style aimed at patient empowerment and physical and psychosocial support. Self-management is also an essential part of patient-centered care. There is a clear link between patient-centered communication and adherence to treatment in mental health care, where a good communicator can double the chance of adherence. Treatment demands vary, and patients differ in their ability to deal with them, the options available to them, and environmental factors. Nurses encourage self-management by providing patients and their families with the right support to manage their own health and quality of life. The success of treatment depends on the expertise of the healthcare professional and the extent to which the patient adheres to the advice and recommendations associated with the treatment. Self-management deficits and self-care deficits may arise if patients are unable to carry out self-management in a targeted manner.

17.4 Patient-Centered Shared Decision-Making

Patient-centered care requires healthcare professionals to adopt an individualized and holistic, biopsychosocial approach to patient management. This is about the patient's illness, but also about improving his health status. By using a communication style aimed at patient empowerment and offering physical and psychosocial support, patient management is stimulated. In line with this, patient-centered care also includes providing self-management support, with the aim that the patient of client will adopt new behavior (for example, exercise more) or change existing behavior (for example, take more rest). To achieve this, you must start from personal preferences and aspects that enable patients to change their behavior. The starting point is shared decision-making (Lawford et al. 2019; Sassen 2023).

There is a clear link between patient-centered communication and adherence to treatment in mental health care. The chance of adherence to treatment is twice as high if the professional is a good communicator. Professionals who are friendly explain the use and purpose of prescribed medication, answer questions and address patient concerns, and discuss treatment aspects (such as medication instructions) to promote their clients' compliance. Medication specific discussion may improve adherence, but an optimistic attitude of professionals also improves patient adherence (Thompson and McCabe 2012; Sassen 2023).

Every treatment has a certain appeal to the patient. Treatment varies and the demands placed on the patient regarding symptom management and self-management also vary. The desired self-management and health behaviors can be relatively simple and relate to familiar behaviors. Taking medication, for example, can be experienced as relatively easy by a patient once a day: it is relatively easy to incorporate into the daily lifestyle. However, it can also be complex and demand new behavior from the patient. For example, it is not easy for people with type 1 diabetes to perform the sequential actions around determining blood sugar value, administering insulin, and eating food in the right way and at the right time. Some treatments require one type of behavior from the patient, while others require several different, multiple behaviors. Treatment can require a change in behavior from the patient for a short to long term.

Patients differ in the extent to which they can deal with this, in the options available to them and in terms of environmental factors. Adherence would therefore be better understood if it was seen as a process of a patient's efforts throughout the disease process to appropriately engage in desired self-management and symptom management behaviors.

Nursing professionals promote self-management by providing patients and their families with the right support to manage their own health and quality of life, with the aim of improving their well-being and patient satisfaction.

In this initial situation, it is important that patients are given an active role in the whole of integrated (preventive and curative) care. They will then be more likely to take an active role regarding their own health. If patients experience the interaction as patient-centered, if healthcare professionals give them the feeling that they are expected to play an active role, the chance increases that they will participate in active and assertive decision-making. They are more open to self-management and the associated desired changes in their lifestyle and health behavior. The patient can then become an active, directing patient or client within the productive interaction with the healthcare professional (Sassen 2023).

Optimizing health outcomes for both the patient at the individual level and at the level of the population is only possible through the combination of effective treatment and treatment follow-up. Follow-up of the treatment by desired behavior (self-management and lifestyle factors) and adherence to therapy. Think of following medication instructions in case of depressive complaints, asthma, cardiac arrhythmias, or high blood pressure. The success of the treatment depends on the expertise of the healthcare professional, but also on the extent to which the person with depressive symptoms, asthma, cardiac arrhythmias, or high blood pressure takes the treatment advice to heart and incorporates it into their health behavior. The best, most effective treatment can turn into an ineffective treatment by not following the desired treatment-related recommendations.

If treatment requires appropriate medication intake, making and keeping appointments, or managing the onset, prognosis, or persistence of the health problem, the success of treatment often depends on compliance. The burden of illness has shifted to chronic health problems, making it more urgent than it was in the past to adhere to desirable precepts to improve the effectiveness of care and treatment. The extent to which people with a health problem adhere decreases as the duration and complexity of the treatment regimen increase. Long-term and complex care and treatment are often inextricably linked to chronic health problems (WHO 2003).

In healthcare, the goal is to provide targeted care and to work toward optimal health outcomes, also referred to as patient outcomes. A patient outcome is the result of the treatment or care. This is influenced by two factors (WHO 2003):

- The first factor is effective treatment.
- The second factor is the extent to which the patient can comply with the advice and recommendations associated with the treatment as agreed.

Whether a patient succeeds in this depends to a large extent on his capacity for self-management and symptom management. This involves bringing and keeping his lifestyle and health behavior in line with what is desirable given his health situation. The patient's symptom management and self-management affect the prognosis.

A patient with renal impairment undergoes a surgical procedure that has been shown to be effective, and a new kidney is placed. This treatment also includes taking medicines to prevent rejection reactions, among other things. From the patient's perspective, this involves both undergoing the procedure and keeping to the associated agreements, in this case taking medication. A patient who suffers from chronic depression is offered treatment from mental health care services in the form of periodic (4 times a year) appointments. In the case of a depressive episode, the intensity is increased according to the severity of the health complaints. For the desired patient outcome, it is crucial that this patient keeps his appointments with the mental health care service, takes his medication, keeps his day-night rhythm regular, and is sufficiently physically active. The success of the treatment, however good it may be, is largely determined by the patient's health behavior.

If patients are unable to carry out self-management in a targeted manner, self-management deficits and self-care deficits may arise. This appears to occur more than average when several healthcare professionals are present around one patient, all of whom work from their own expertise and who call in each other if a problem exceeds their own expertise and/or responsibility. If, in such a case, the patient is insufficiently able to take control of his own health and cannot direct the care, it is up to the nurse to inhibit that each healthcare professional only covers part of the care circle and that there is no coordination in healthcare. Each healthcare professional then has its own range of care and treatment, but there is no direction. Nurses can play an important role by standing next to the patient and supporting the patient's control function or ensuring that it is restored (Fig. 17.1). The self-management and self-care deficits can be remedied, thanks to nursing input.

Disease management is about supporting the patient in self-management and lifestyle management. It covers the entire care pathway:

- disease prevention;
- early disease detection;
- reducing symptoms of the health problem;
- prevention of worsening of symptoms;
- the promotion of optimal self-management of the health situation;
- encouraging a lifestyle and health behavior that can have a beneficial effect on the health situation.

Self-management is an important perspective on care for nurses. Self-management is the favorable treatment of one's own health as far as people are able to do it themselves. Self-management support and self-management promotion therefore

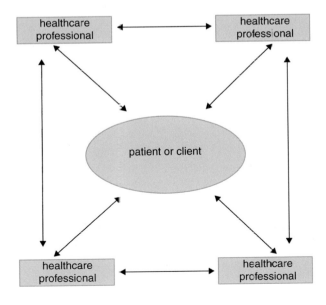

Fig. 17.1 Relationship between patient, self-management and health (beeldrechten: [rechten bij auteur] bestand:)

require customization: one person may need much more support and explanation than the other in order to deal with this own health and to make his health status as favorably as possible.

The word self-management indicates that the care should be aimed at (restoring) one's own control. The patient must do it himself, to manage his own health—or rather to be the manager of his life—even if he has a health problem. The point of departure for nurses must be that they provide self-management support, support, where this is (temporarily) necessary. The patient learns to get started with his self-management, but if that fails (temporarily, with episodes, more long-term), the nurse provides self-management support that is tailored to the patient's needs and the need to provide care. Self-management support is aimed at improving the quality of care. Self-management promotion is self-management support.

Promoting patient self-management requires nursing professionals to demonstrate a commitment to the importance of health promotion and prevention. This commitment is vital for creating more focus on health promotion and prevention in patient care. This commitment applies to all healthcare professionals, so that opportunities for a healthier society are created. Because although it is known that the impact of chronic health problems can be reduced with targeted prevention and health promotion, little attention and budget are devoted to this in the health care sector.

Our health care system barely focuses on keeping people healthy, on prevention, and on health promotion. A large part of the attention and the budget is devoted to acute care. The focus is on specialist, technically complicated care, while much health gain can be expected if the principles of disease prevention and health promotion were better applied within nursing care. For nursing professionals, health promotion and prevention should be an integral part of every patient contact, with the aim of promoting health based on patient needs and expanding it where possible. This can and will be successful if the focus is on supporting the balance in maintaining health and promoting and optimizing the quality of life and life expectancy (Sassen 2023).

The number of people with chronic diseases is still increasing and this largely determines the burden of disease in the population. The number of people whose well-being is affected by not one but several health problems at the same time is also increasing. This multimorbidity adversely affects the burden of disease in the population. For patients with a high burden of disease, the search for and provision of the right care and treatment often cause a disruption in daily life. These patients are confronted with all kinds of recommendations and things they should or should not do. From the perspective of healthcare professionals, these recommendations are a logical consequence of care and treatment: if patients would adopt these recommendations, this would have a beneficial effect on care and treatment. In practice, however, it appears that the extent to which patients adopt all advice and recommendations as agreed with the healthcare professional is far from optimal (WHO 2003). And that is not surprising if we take a critical look at how the recommendations are applied in care and treatment. We first look at this from the perspective of the nursing professionals and other healthcare professionals, and then we look at it from the perspective of patients and clients.

1. From the perspective of healthcare professionals, these are the recommendations that are seen as necessary if care and treatment are to be efficient and effective. Healthcare professionals provide targeted care and treatment that is tailored to the patient. This makes sense from their perspective, patient come to receive efficient and effective, evidence-based care and treatment. Their assumption is that the associated recommendations and advice are implemented by the patient. The most common intervention that is carried out by healthcare professionals to realize the 'being done of the recommendations and advices' is information provision. The healthcare professional informs the patient, gives his recommendations to the patient, and expects the patient to adopt these recommendations.

   Patient management (both in terms of care and treatment) is also about promoting patient self-management. Promoting the patient's self-management is important because care and treatment often require that patients start with behavioral and/or lifestyle advice from the moment they become ill and maintain this for the duration of their illness. Patient-centered care can provide the patient with targeted support as he starts to master self-management, but this process is not always smooth. Professionals do not use a person-centered way of communicating to the patient.

   Communication between professionals and patients is often professional-centered, with the relationship being determined by the healthcare professional's agenda (Lawford et al. 2019).

2. If we look from the perspective of the patient and clients, it turns out that they have a different view on the extent to which recommendations should be followed. It appears that the patient's amount of knowledge is not directly related to whether or not he 'follows' the recommendations (WHO 2003).

   The combination of disease burden and unfavorable treatment adherence is a cause for concern—especially if we know that the risk of non-adherence increases with the duration and complexity of treatment, as is the case with chronic health problems and with multimorbidity.

   The nursing intervention information provision is often experienced by patients as something they already know, as information about patients in general and as information not about themselves specifically.

   Important factors such as the patient's view of their own disease and symptoms and the recommendations received are usually only taken into account to a limited extent.

   The biomedical model of health and disease remains a fairly dominant perspective in health care. This biomedical perspective assumes that patients more or less passively adopt the recommendations of healthcare professionals, but patients do not share this perspective (WHO 2003).

What may be the solution to dilute the perspectives? A meta-review shows that interventions that are tailored to the unique situation of the patient, in which both self-management support and emotional support are offered at the same time, lead to patient-centered care (Naef et al. 2019). An important element of patient-centered care is the promotion of the patient's self-management, self-management promotion, and the promotion of healthy lifestyles to optimize health status and quality of life (Sassen 2023).

While information provision rarely leads to lifestyle and behavioral change or to better self-management and patient management, we do know that the systematic use of a collaborative process with the patient can be effective for lifestyle or behavior change. We also know how we as healthcare professionals can systematically direct behavior change (Sassen 2023):

- A process of behavior change starts with discussing the patient's perception of his individual risk of (worsening) the health problem and/or the associated risk factors. This is about risk-perception.
- Subsequently, the advantages and disadvantages should be discussed, so that the patient can consider whether a change in his lifestyle or self-management behavior is a good personal choice for him. This is about decisional balance.
- The next of kin can offer the patient social support in optimizing his lifestyle and self-management behavior and to look for (long-term) social support and discuss how the patient can deal with social pressure. This is about handling social situations in regard to self-management and lifestyle management.
- If the intended patient management requires specific skills, you should work with the patient to see how he can master these skills. These skills are needed to realize the self-management of lifestyle behavior. Patient management can best be specified in an action plan with a description of the when-where-and-how. This action plan supports the patient or client in behavior change.
- If the action plan is combined with a coping plan, the change in behavior can be converted into behavior maintenance. Maintenance can be difficult because high-risk situations can withheld the person from the self-management or lifestyle behavior. Using a coping plan can help to prevent relapse (Sassen 2023).

17.5 Conclusion

- Patient-centered care is a crucial approach in healthcare that aims to optimize health outcomes for patients. It involves empowering patients through effective communication, providing support, and promoting self-management. This approach, coupled with patient's compliance, is essential in achieving the desired health outcomes.
- Adherence to the recommended treatment plan is essential, and healthcare professionals play a vital role in ensuring patients are compliant. By embracing this approach, healthcare professionals can provide targeted care that works toward optimal health outcomes for both the patient at an individual level and at the level of the population.

- The aim of disease management is to provide high-quality care by empowering patients to take control of their health through self-management support and health promotion.
- Although healthcare professionals have an important role in promoting patient self-management, patient-centered communication is necessary for successful implementation of healthcare advice and recommendations.
- A shift toward health promotion and prevention in the healthcare sector could have a significant impact on the burden of disease in the population, particularly for patients with multiple health problems. Therefore, it is essential to increase the focus on health promotion and prevention in patient care and improve the quality of life and life expectancy for patients.

Box 17.1 Mind-Map Patient Management
Create a mind-map on the importance of patient-centered care in healthcare.

Point out how healthcare professionals need to adopt an individualized and holistic, biopsychosocial approach to patient management to improve the patient's health and well-being.

Use: Highlight the importance of communication and patient empowerment, self-management, shared decision-making, and physical and psychosocial support to stimulate patient management.

Box 17.2 Mind-Map Patient-Centered Communication and Adherence
Create a mind-map on adherence to treatment in mental health care.

Point out the link between patient-centered communication and adherence to treatment in mental health care.

Use: The importance of healthcare professionals being friendly, explaining medication use and purpose, answering questions and addressing patient concerns, discussing treatment aspects, and promoting medication-specific discussion to improve adherence.

Box 17.3 Mind-Map Self-Management and Symptom Management
Create a mind-map on self-management and symptom management.

Point out the importance of self-management and symptom management in healthcare and how it affects treatment outcomes.

Highlights the need for patients (to comply with advice and recommendations associated with treatment, incorporate desirable lifestyle and health behaviors, and manage their symptoms to achieve optimal health outcomes) vs. the need for healthcare professionals.

Box 17.4 Mind-Map Commitment to Health Promotion and Disease Prevention
Make a mind-map on commitment to health promotion and disease prevention.
   Put the patient at the center of the mind-map.
   Commitment to health promotion and prevention means that you as a healthcare professional … [indicate the actions], with the aim of promoting self-management of the patient to achieve better health and quality of life.

Box 17.5 Mind-Map Optimal Patient Management and Self-Management
Make a mind-map and focus on optimal patient management and self-management.
   Place on the left the barriers that can impede the optimization of patient management and patient self-management, from the perspective of healthcare professionals.
   Place on the right the opportunities that optimizing patient management and self-management offers the patient, seen from the patient's perspective.
   Highlight what is important to you.

Nursing and Patient-Centered Communication

18

18.1 Topic List

1. Importance of effective communication in building a relationship of trust between healthcare professionals and patients/clients.
2. Verbal and non-verbal communication in the process of exchange between healthcare professionals and patients/clients.
3. Key functions of communication in patient-centered care, including ensuring a positive relationship, addressing patient needs, responding to patient emotions, facilitating informed and shared decision-making, and promoting healthy lifestyle and self-management.
4. Specific communication skills for different functions of communication in patient-centered care.
5. Relationship between patient satisfaction and verbal communication, including involvement and support from healthcare professionals.
6. Role of non-verbal communication in patient satisfaction, including facial expression, pose, tone of voice, and proximity.
7. Characteristics of an effective interaction style of healthcare professionals, including affective connection, shared control, and negotiating options.
8. Importance of active listening in building a cooperative relationship with patients/clients, including reflecting, summarizing, introducing silences, paraphrasing, and non-verbal encouragement.
9. The need for respectful care, including responding to patient values and standards, acting in a caring and compassionate manner, and treating patients and families with respect and without prejudice.
10. Balancing the biomedical and communicative perspectives on care and treatment, and the positive effects of optimizing the communicative perspective on patient satisfaction and adherence to recommendations.

18.2   Introduction

Effective communication is essential in building a trusting relationship between healthcare professionals and patients. Active listening, empathy, and the exchange of verbal and non-verbal communication are key components in patient-centered care. This communication helps to ensure a positive relationship, respond to the patient's emotions, and enable informed decision-making. Furthermore, optimizing the communicative perspective on care and treatment has a positive effect on patient satisfaction and on patient management.

18.3   Topics

This chapter focuses on the importance of effective communication in building a relationship of trust between healthcare professionals and patients, which is necessary for patient-centered care. The author discusses the key functions of communication between patient and nursing professional, such as ensuring a positive relationship, responding to the patient's emotions, and enabling the patient to adopt a healthy lifestyle. The chapter highlights the specific communication skills required for each function, such as active listening and exploring issues that concern the patient or client. The passage also explores the relationship between patient satisfaction and verbal and non-verbal communication, with specific communicative factors that lead to patient satisfaction. The author emphasizes the importance of respectful care and adopting a committed and friendly communication style. Finally, the chapter discusses the limitations of the communicative perspective alone in ensuring that patients adopt recommendations in their daily lives, suggesting that it needs to be embedded in a larger whole of respectful care.

18.4   Effective Interaction with Patients and Clients

Every professional can build a relationship of trust with the patient or client through effective communication, an important condition for patient-centered care. You do this by listening actively, from a calm, especially unhurried attitude (Lor et al. 2016).

For effective communication, a continuous process of exchange of verbal and non-verbal communication between the patient and the healthcare professional is important. The professional is expected to adopt a reflective and listening attitude, in which the professional radiates empathy and involvement to the patient and recognizes and understands the patient's non-verbal communication and feelings. Non-verbal expressions of communication are eye contact, gestures, and facial expressions. Verbal communication is what is said in spoken language, including tone and intonation (Lor et al. 2016).

There are a number of key functions of (verbal and non-verbal) communication between patient and healthcare professional (Levinson et al. 2010):

– ensuring a positive relationship;
– communicating with attention to what the patient needs and/or wants;
– communication that responds to patient's emotions;
– communication aimed at informed and shared decision-making;
– communication aimed at enabling the patient to adopt a healthy lifestyle, self-management, and symptom management.

Each of these functions requires a specific set of communication skills (Levinson et al. 2010). For example, communicating with attention to what patients need and wishes requires exploring issues that concern the patient, about what has priority and what the patient thinks is important. The professional should listen to the patient's answers and ask follow-up questions if the answer needs to be clarified. For example, communicating about decision-making calls for discussing realistic expectations about care and treatment and correcting and discussing unrealistic expectations.

A systematic review with meta-analysis revealed a relationship between patient satisfaction and verbal communication (Oliveira et al. 2012). Communication that demonstrates the involvement of the healthcare professional increases the level of patient satisfaction. The same applies to communication in which patients are offered support. Linked to the non-verbal communication, the time spent reading the patient's record was another factor that promoted patient satisfaction.

Patient satisfaction mainly depends on the quality of the interaction with the patient. Other factors that play a role are the quality of the treatment or care and the satisfaction with the clinical outcomes after treatment (Oliveira et al. 2012).

Specific communicative factors that lead to patient satisfaction for verbal communication are a psychosocially oriented conversation content; that expresses empathy from the words; and that the words are comforting. For non-verbal communication, communicative factors that lead to patient satisfaction are: facial expression; pose; tone of voice, and close proximity.

The interaction style of the professional is characterized by an affective connection and openness to the patient, sharing control over the conduct of the conversation and negotiating options (Oliveira et al. 2012).

Active listening by healthcare professionals offers many opportunities to build a good cooperative relationship with the patient. Active listening is about reflecting on what the patient is saying ("You sound very disappointed that you have been uncertain about the results of the tests you have had for so long"). Active listening is also about summarizing what the patient is saying ("Before we move on, I would like to look back with you on the past period and what you have achieved so far"). Active listening is also introducing silences into the conversation, encouraging the patient to collect his own thoughts before continuing to talk. Active listening is also paraphrasing, such as when a patient says he wants to stop treatment ("It sounds like you are saying that the illness is driving you to despair"). Active listening also means non-verbally encouraging the patient to tell his story by nodding, smiling invitingly or responding with "mmmm" or "ooohh" (Arnold and Underman Boggs 2020).

Despite the huge improvements it offers in patient care and treatment, the communicative perspective alone is not enough to ensure that patients adopt recommendations in their daily lives. To achieve this, attentive and empathetic communication needs to be embedded in a larger whole of respectful care.

Providing respectful care is about responding to and accepting the values and standards of the patient. Respectful care is also about acting in a caring, sympathetic, courteous, and positive manner. It means that the patient and his family are treated with an open mind, without prejudice, even if their values and standards differ from your own. Respectful interaction with patient and family has been characterized as sensitive and with compassion (Lor et al. 2016).

If we try to let go of the biomedical perspective on care, a communicative perspective can get more space for nursing professionals. From a communicative perspective, the emphasis is on developing good communication skills and working toward a more equal relationship between the nursing professional and the patient. Optimizing the communicative perspective on care and treatment has a positive effect on patient's satisfaction with the care and treatment offered. It is necessary for nurses to adopt a committed and friendly communication style.

While the biomedical perspective on care and treatment does not sufficiently support the patient applying the recommendations, the communicative perspective alone is also insufficient to ensure that patients adopt recommendations in their daily lives.

18.5   Conclusion

- Effective communication is a key component of patient-centered care and involves a continuous process of verbal and non-verbal exchange between healthcare professionals and patients.
- It requires healthcare professionals to adopt a reflective and listening attitude, radiate empathy, and involvement and recognize and understand patients' non-verbal communication and feelings.
- The key functions of communication between healthcare professionals and patients include ensuring a positive relationship, responding to patient emotions, informed and shared decision-making, and enabling patients to adopt a healthy lifestyle and self-management.
- Active listening is essential for building a good cooperative relationship with the patient, which leads to better patient satisfaction.
- Respectful care is necessary for patients to adopt recommendations in their daily lives. While the communicative perspective alone is not enough, optimizing communication skills and developing a committed and friendly communication style can positively impact patient satisfaction with care and treatment.

Box 18.1 Mind-Map Building a Relationship of Trust

Create a mind-map about the importance of effective communication in building a relationship of trust between healthcare professionals and patients or clients.

Point out key functions of communication between healthcare professionals and patients, such as ensuring a positive relationship, responding to the patient's emotions, and enabling decision-making.

Point out what healthcare professionals need to do for that, such as to adopt a committed and friendly communication style, and active listening.

Box 18.2 Mind-Map Facets of Communication

Make a mind-map and place the patient on the left, communication in the middle and the healthcare professional on the right. Organize what happens using the following facets of communication (adapted from Watzlawick 2011):

1. All communication is communication, you cannot not not communicate.
2. All communication has both a content and a relationship level.
3. Communication is the exchange of messages between communicating persons.
4. Communication can take place in an active and a passive manner.
5. Relations within communication can be symmetrical (interaction is characterized by equality and minimal difference) or complementary (interaction is characterized by difference).

Nursing and Narrative Approach

19

19.1 Topic List

1. The Importance of Personal Narratives in Patient-Centered, Relationship-Based Nursing.
2. Understanding the Patient's Personality through Personal Narratives.
3. The Process of Co-Creating Narratives in Patient Interviews.
4. The Healing Power of Personal Narratives in Patient Care.
5. Personal Growth and Meaning-Making through Narratives in Healthcare.
6. Shifting Focus from Diagnoses to Life Stories in Patient Care.
7. Understanding Patients Better through Narratives in Mental Health Care.
8. Using Narratives to Understand the Lives of Older Adults in Geriatric Care.
9. Challenges of Being a Patient and Factors Affecting Patient Well-Being.
10. Key Behaviors of Healthcare Professionals and Their Impact on Patient Outcomes.
11. Partnership in the Nurse-Patient Relationship: Discussing Treatment Options and Lifestyle Changes.
12. The Positive Effect of Nurse Communication Style on Patient Well-Being in Care and Treatment.

19.2 Introduction

Narratives are an important tool for patient-centered, relationship-based nursing, allowing nursing professional to understand a patient's personality and build a relationship of trust. Personal narratives provide meaning to memories and can have a therapeutic effect on patients, leading to personal growth and a more positive self-image. The co-creation of narratives with patients allows for a deeper understanding of their lives and can lead to new insights. Patient-related factors, healthcare system-related factors, and key behaviors of healthcare professionals all play a role in

B. Sassen, *Improving Person-Centered Innovation of Nursing Care*, https://doi.org/10.1007/978-3-031-35048-1_19

making it easier for patients to navigate the healthcare system. For nurses, understanding the patient's history and building a partnership with the patient are important aspects of providing quality care. Ultimately, a positive communication style can have a significant impact on the patient's well-being and perceived quality of life.

19.3 Topics

This chapter is about how personal narratives can be used in nursing care to understand patients better and improve their care. The text explains that patients' personal stories are essential to building relationships of trust. The text also explains how co-creating narratives can give meaning to their memories and experiences. These narratives can help patients to better understand their lives, gain a better view of the future, and even lead to personal growth. The chapter also discusses the challenges faced by patients, including disease complexity, uncertainty, and feelings of isolation or alienation. The role of healthcare professionals, particularly nurses, is also explored, with a focus on effective communication, patient-specific information, and partnership-based care. Finally, the text concludes by emphasizing the importance of empathy, intuition, and reflection in supporting patients' personal narratives and well-being.

19.4 Patients' Personal Narratives

For patient-centered, relationship-based nursing, narratives can be a way of understanding a patient's personality. A personal narrative is an autobiographical story built on life events. The way in which the patient or client tells the story is important here. Most patients start with less emotional aspects and the life events are linked by the patient. Because of this, these life events take on a deeper meaning.

Patient interview would provide the opportunity for the patient to tell their unique, own (life) story, thereby building trust, elucidating symptoms and concerns, elucidating biopsychosocial aspects in the context of life, and building a relationship of trust (Morgan and Yoder 2012).

Narratives can lead to the unfolding of one's life and are also called life journey or life history (Gaydos 2005).

The function of personal narratives is that they can give meaning to memories of the patient and that this can have a function within the care provision. Narratives are created in a process of co-creation. On the basis of memories, the patient talks about events from his past. Together with the nurse, the patient constructs a narrative from this, a story. This experience, describing how events happened in the past and stitching it together into a story, can be experienced as healing by the patient. The idea is also that narratives can lead to personal growth (Gaydos 2005).

Each interaction that involves co-creation is unique and can lead to new insights. When the patient's story is heard, the patient's memories are understood in a different way. This allows the story to be confirmed: it is given meaning. Patients may be able to understand their lives better and gain a better view of the future. For example, a narrative can help a patient not to feel victimized by living conditions, but rather to arrive at a more positive self-image (Gaydos 2005).

Narratives provide professionals with tools to understand patients better, so that the patient can also feel better understood. This form of—sometimes very profound—personal communication offers a shift from focusing on diagnoses and interventions, to giving meaning to someone's life story with all its peaks and valleys. For professionals, intuition is important here, apart from an empathetic, reflective attitude that supports the patient in telling his personal narrative (Gaydos 2005).

As a nurse, it is good to look at and understand the patient's history. Personal narratives are certainly important in mental health care as it creates opportunities for recovery and offers hope as old narratives are rewritten and new narratives (for the future) are visualized (Gaydos 2005). Narratives in gerontology, in the care of people at an advanced age or with more serious chronic health problems, help to understand how life went, how life was lived by the patient (Kenyon 2015).

Being a patient is not easy, but what factors make it difficult for people? Due to a disease, people are confronted with the complexity of having to live with a health problem. Life gets turned upside down because of this. People are also faced with uncertainty regarding the duration of the health problem. Characteristics of the health problem can be difficult for the patient and even lead to a person feeling alienated from themselves. The patient can feel abandoned by his illness, he can feel overwhelmed, he can lose all confidence in his own body, but also confidence in his own abilities or mental abilities. The patient may feel socially isolated or misunderstood by his environment. Treatment can be accompanied by iatrogenic effects, which present the patient with new problems or exacerbation of existing problems. The cost of illness is also an important factor for many people.

In addition to the intrinsic factors mentioned, there are also factors outside the patient that can take their toll. Characteristics of the healthcare system have an influence, as waiting lists, appointments that do not match, consultations with several healthcare professionals. The interaction with (several) healthcare professionals can cause problems for the patient. After all, communicating with healthcare professionals is a lot more difficult if you are concerned about your health, if you do not (yet) know what is going on, but you are already expected to think along about your own illness.

Being a patient is not easy, but there are several specific tools to better deal with this. Firstly, these are "key behaviors" of healthcare professionals and factors related to the healthcare system and secondly, patient-related factors (WHO 2003).

1. Key-behaviors of healthcare professionals and factors related to the healthcare system. The healthcare professional prescribes a particular treatment regimen. This is done based on guidelines, protocols or 'best practice' care provision. They choose the treatment that best suits the individual patient in front of them, monitor the clinical outcomes and provide feedback to the patient on all kinds of

issues related to the treatment. The way healthcare professionals communicate with their patients and interact with the individual patient has an important influence on the patient and how they feel, move, and behave in the healthcare system. The way of interaction and communication strongly influences the patient's feeling of well-being, his perceived quality of life and ultimately also the patient outcomes.

What can guide the care and treatment relationship of nurses? The following aspects provide insight into a relationship with the patient that involves partnership. A partnership exists when:

(a) there is support to discuss treatment options;
(b) "negotiation" is possible about the treatment regime;
(c) there may be discussion about whether or not to adopt—and wholly or partly—the lifestyle changes or self-management behaviors that result from or are appropriate to the treatment regime.

The communication style of the nurse has a positive effect on the patient's well-being. Your communication style is experienced as positive by the patient if you provide patient-specific, individual-oriented information, ask patient-specific questions (appropriate to their care and treatment), and if you talk positively. If clarity is provided about the diagnosis and treatment, this is perceived as pleasant by the patient, especially if there is a chronic health problem. Patients also experience continuity of care and follow-up as pleasant. An empathetic and a "warm," involved attitude on the part of the healthcare professional and a relaxed, calm attitude in which the patient gets the feeling that there is time and space in the agenda of the professional are perceived as important by the patient. It is also important for patients that there is interaction with the healthcare professional, in which both share information, build a relationship together and in which the professional provides emotional support. Patients who are satisfied with their healthcare professional and are satisfied with the treatment regimen are more likely to comply with treatment and care agreements.

If your goal is for the patient to be central to the care and for the patient to feel involved in the care, it is important that communication with the patient is always structured, that it is thought through from the perspective of the patient and that the interaction is professional (not too familiar), and carefully. What we see in professional practice is that healthcare professionals provide information, try to motivate the patient and that they recognize that certain skills are important to enable the patient to improve his health. In practice, however, it appears that healthcare professionals only inform patients sparsely, but have very limited motivational skills and that healthcare professionals also experience a lack of knowledge and even frustration in teaching skills, help them making an action and coping plan etc., while they should motivate them (WHO 2003).

2. Patient and clients related factors. The meaning people give to their experiences, and therefore also to their self-image, is constantly changing. There are indications that this contains important therapeutic potential. Patients are only open to treatment and counseling if it provides a plausible explanation for what

they have been through. For example, in psychotherapy only 15% of the effect could be attributed to the methods and techniques followed, 15% to a placebo effect and the hope and expectation that things will get better, 30% to the personal relationship with the therapist, and more than 40% to the patient's willingness to move (Hubble et al. 1999). This willingness to "move," to change, is largely related to the awareness that patients develop about their situation and condition. The nursing professional can mediate in this by paying attention to a number of essential matters:

(a) What does the patient feel or what does he think is happening to him at this moment?
(b) How does the patient explain what is wrong with him or what is happening to him?
(c) What does the patient think needs to be done?
(d) What examples are there of desired behavior? This may have already occurred in the form of "little miracles," which can serve as a starting point for generalizing to a situation of greater health and well-being for the patient.

The experience of illness and the distress it causes, as well as the care and treatment received, are critical chapters in the patient's life journey.

19.5 Conclusion

- Personal narratives play a crucial role in patient-centered and relationship-based nursing. By understanding the patient's history and partnering with them in their care, nurses can provide quality care and help patients navigate the healthcare system.
- Narratives offer a way for nursing professionals to understand the patient's personality, build trust, and gain insights into the patient's biopsychosocial aspects in the context of their life.
- The co-creation of a patient's narrative with a nursing professional can lead to healing experiences, personal growth, and a better understanding of the patient's life story. Effective communication is essential, and the way healthcare professionals communicate and interact with their patients can significantly impact patient outcomes.
- By focusing on the patient's narrative, healthcare professionals can move away from focusing solely on diagnoses and interventions and instead give meaning to a patient's life story.
- Being a patient or client is not easy, and healthcare professionals must adopt key behaviors and consider patient-related factors to ensure a positive patient outcome.
- Ultimately, by adopting a partnership approach, healthcare professionals can communicate with their patients effectively, leading to better outcomes and a better quality of life for the patient.

Box 19.1 Mind-Map Importance of Personal Narratives

Create a mind-map on the importance of personal narratives in patient-centered nursing.

Point out how narratives can help nurses understand a patient's personality and how this understanding can improve nursing care.

Point out how narratives can optimize the health situation of the patient or client.

Box 19.2 Mind-Map Narrative Approach

Create a mind-map on using a narrative approach.

Point out why a narrative approach to the patient can lead to patient-centered nursing care.

Circle (three) important points for attention.

Nursing and Relationship-Centered Care (RCC)

20

20.1 Topic List: Toward Relationship-Centered Care (RCC)

1. Relationship-Centered Care (RCC): Definition, principles, and goals.
2. Importance of Relationship Skills in Healthcare: Empathy, reflection, and their impact on patient outcomes.
3. RCC at Different Levels: Exploring reciprocal interactions between healthcare professionals and patients, colleagues, and the healthcare system and society.
4. Uniqueness of Nurses in RCC: Their role in supporting high-quality care, working environment, and healthcare system functioning.
5. Positive Health Outcomes of RCC: Adherence, symptom management, clinical and functional improvement, patient loyalty, and decreased malpractice risk.
6. Patient-Centered Care vs. Relationship-Centered Care: Understanding the differences and benefits of RCC.
7. Role of Policies and Procedures in Healthcare System: Aligning with RCC principles to provide appropriate care and treatment.
8. Patient Engagement and Partnership in RCC: Active involvement in care and treatment process for improved well-being and quality of life.
9. Challenges and Barriers to Implementing RCC: Addressing barriers and promoting RCC in healthcare settings.
10. Future Directions of Healthcare: Emphasizing RCC as a key component of high-quality healthcare.

20.2 Introduction

Healthcare is a complex and constantly evolving field, with new treatments and technologies emerging all the time. While these advances are undoubtedly important, it is also crucial to remember the fundamental role that relationships play in

B. Sassen, *Improving Person-Centered Innovation of Nursing Care*, https://doi.org/10.1007/978-3-031-35048-1_20

healthcare. Relationship-centered care (RCC) is an approach that recognizes the importance of empathy, communication, and reflection in delivering high-quality care to patients.

RCC goes beyond patient-centered care by emphasizing reciprocal interactions at the micro, meso, and macro levels in healthcare. Healthcare has been constantly changing to provide higher quality, more evidence-based care and treatment.

With the focus on patient-centered care, healthcare professionals have been able to understand the importance of putting the patient's needs and preferences at the forefront of their care.

However, relationship-centered care (RCC) takes this a step further by recognizing the importance of the relationships that you as a nurse have with your patients, your multidisciplinary team of colleagues, and as being part of the healthcare system. RCC emphasizes the importance of reciprocal interactions at different levels of healthcare, ultimately resulting in improved patient outcomes.

20.3 Topics

This chapter revolves around the concept of relationship-centered care (RCC) in healthcare and highlights the importance of relationship skills such as empathy and reflection in improving patient outcomes of care. RCC goes beyond patient-centered care by focusing on reciprocal interactions at micro, meso, and macro levels in healthcare. The chapter explains that RCC is about the relationship of the healthcare professional with the patient (micro-level), with colleagues (meso-level), and with the healthcare system and society (macro-level). The importance and uniqueness of every nurse in relation to others are emphasized, and the article highlights how a good relationship between the nurse and the patient leads to positive health outcomes, including higher adherence, improved clinical and functional status, patient loyalty, and fewer errors. Furthermore, the chapter explains that the healthcare system is designed to work toward high-quality healthcare. The policies and procedures in place are intended to provide appropriate care and treatment for one or more patient health problems. If the patient feels like a partner in the cooperative relationship with the nurse and is actively involved in the care process, this will lead to better patient outcomes and improved quality of life. Overall, the content in this topic underscores the importance of relationship-centered care in healthcare and how it can positively impact patient outcomes and well-being.

20.4 Relationship-Centered Patient Care

Healthcare should evolve toward relationship-centered care (RCC). Relationship skills, such as empathy and reflection, improve patient outcomes of care. RCC goes beyond patient-centered care by focusing on reciprocal interactions at the micro, meso, and macro levels in healthcare.

RCC is about the relationship of the healthcare professional with the patient (micro-level), with his or her colleagues (meso-level), and with the healthcare system and society (macro-level) (Weiss and Swede 2019).

Relationship-centered care is about the importance and uniqueness of every nurse in relation to others. In these relationships, the nurse supports a high quality of care, a high-quality working environment, and the high-quality functioning of the health care system. A good relationship between the nursing professional and the patient leads to positive health outcomes. Among other things, it leads to a higher degree of adherence, a decrease in symptoms, an improvement in clinical and functional status, but also more patient loyalty and fewer errors (malpractice risk) (Weiss and Swede 2019).

The healthcare system is designed to work toward high-quality healthcare. The policies and procedures in place in the health care system are intended to provide appropriate care and treatment for one or more patient health problems.

If the patient feels like a partner in the cooperative relationship with the nurse and if they feel actively involved in the care and treatment process, this will lead to a better well-being of the patient and a better quality of life. This also improves positive health outcomes and positive patient outcomes.

20.5 Conclusion

- RCC is an important approach that healthcare professionals should adopt to provide better care and treatment to their patients and clients.
- By focusing on building strong relationships with patients, colleagues, and the healthcare system, healthcare professionals can create a cooperative environment that fosters high-quality care and improved patient outcomes.
- The importance of empathy and reflection in healthcare cannot be overstated, and RCC recognizes this by prioritizing the relationships that healthcare professionals have.
- The shift toward relationship-centered care (RCC) is a crucial step for healthcare professionals and organizations to take. By prioritizing empathy, reflection, and communication skills, healthcare professionals can create strong, cooperative relationships with patients, colleagues, and the healthcare system, leading to improved patient outcomes and greater patient loyalty.
- RCC recognizes the importance of reciprocal interactions at all levels of healthcare and fosters a high-quality working environment for healthcare professionals. RCC should be a core focus of healthcare organizations, and investment in training and resources to support this approach will benefit both patients and healthcare professionals.
- By embracing RCC, healthcare can move toward a more patient-centered, relationship-based approach that prioritizes positive health outcomes and improves the overall quality of care.

Box 20.1 Mind-Map Positive Characteristics of Relationship-Centered Nursing Care

Create a mind-map on the positive characteristics of relationship-centered nursing care.

Point out the positive characteristics of relationship-centered nursing care at the micro-, meso- and macro-level.

Point out for each level (micro-, meso- and macro-level) what you should do/think of/use as a nursing professional.

What is the added value of this compared to patient-centered care for nursing professionals?

Nursing and Integrated Care

21

21.1 Topic List for Integrated Care and Its Benefits

1. Definition of integrated care: Understanding the concept of integrated care.
2. Improved accessibility of healthcare services, particularly those with complex health problems and multimorbidity.
3. Enhanced quality of healthcare services by coordinating care between professionals, organizations, and sectors, and focusing on patient needs and preferences.
4. Integrated care can improve continuity of care by establishing collaborative relationships between patients and healthcare professionals.
5. Integrated care is centered on the needs and preferences of the patient, involving them in the care and treatment decision-making process.
6. Importance of effective communication between healthcare professionals and patients in integrated care, including frequent contact, information sharing, and involving patients in the care process.
7. Impact of reimbursement systems on integrated care, and the need for aligning reimbursement with patient needs and preferences.
8. Challenges and limitations of integrated care.
9. Comparison integrated care with specialized and differentiated care, highlighting the risks of fragmentation of care and lower quality of care.
10. Conceptual model of integrated care, including clinical integration at the micro-level, meso-level, and macro-level.
11. Exploring integrated care and complementary health care to provide patient-centered care.

21.2   Introduction

Integrated care is a healthcare approach that interweaves different facilities to create integrated healthcare systems that provide improved accessibility, quality, and continuity of services to patients. The goal of integrated care is to optimize care and treatment by combining parts so that they work together to form a whole. Patient satisfaction can increase if they have more frequent contact with healthcare professionals, access to information sharing, and continuity of care. The healthcare system has a limited availability of resources, which may result in increased demand and pressure on healthcare professionals.

Integrated care is a model that focuses on integrating, connecting, and coordinating care for patients on micro, meso, and macro levels. At the micro-level, clinical integration is about coordinating care between professionals and across institutional and sectoral boundaries. At the meso-level, organizations and professional partnerships integrate to provide cohesive and coordinated care. At the macro-level, partnerships are formed between organizations to create a care continuum that is patient centered. Integrated care aims to eliminate duplication of information and tests and combine approaches from regular and alternative, complementary healthcare.

21.3   Topics

This chapter discusses integrated care and its importance in improving healthcare services. Integrated care refers to the interweaving of healthcare facilities to create integrated healthcare systems that improve accessibility, quality, and continuity of services. The passage discusses several factors that influence the quality of care, including the way in which appointments are made, the frequency of contact between healthcare professionals and patients, the sharing of information between healthcare facilities, continuity of care, the reimbursement system in health care, and the limited availability of resources.

The chapter also emphasizes that integrated care is diametrically opposed to specialized and differentiated care, which can lead to fragmentation of care and lower quality of care. It describes a conceptual model that can be used to make integrated care transparent. This model is divided into micro, meso, and macro levels, with a focus on coordinating care between professionals and organizations to improve efficiency and quality of care. Finally, the passage discusses the importance of integrative medicine, which combines approaches from both regular and alternative, complementary health care to provide patient-centered care.

21.4 Integrated Patient Care

Integrated care is about "linking" healthcare facilities. The integrated healthcare systems thus created can improve the accessibility, quality, and continuity of health care services. These integrated healthcare systems make it possible to better tailor care to the patient, and this certainly applies to patients with complex health problems and multimorbidity (Valentijn et al. 2013).

Goodwin (2013) defines integrated care as follows:

"a simple idea-combining parts so that they work to form a whole in order to optimize care and treatment."

The healthcare system influences the patient and the way in which it is possible for the patient to navigate the healthcare system.

- A first factor that influences the patient is the way in which an appointment can be made for a contact moment, the length and duration of a treatment and specifically the details of the contact moment between patient and healthcare professional. Healthcare professionals indicate that there is often insufficient time to properly discuss what is desired with the patient. And that the lack of time applies specifically to topics related to desirable lifestyle changes, such as patient symptom management and self-management.
- A second factor is that the health care system determines to what extent healthcare professionals can communicate with the patient. If more frequent contact is possible (telephone contact with concerns or questions, or to pass on and discuss the results of a diagnostic test or examination), this keeps the patient more involved in the care and treatment. This simple and cost-effective way of communicating with patients often also has a beneficial effect on the patient's symptom management and self-management behavior.
- A third factor is the way healthcare facilities share information. On the one hand, this concerns the sharing of information with the patient, so that he has insight into his file, and on the other hand, it concerns the exchange of information between healthcare professionals.
- A fourth factor is that healthcare determines the continuity of care. Patient satisfaction appears to increase if someone keeps in contact with the same healthcare professional and a collaborative relationship is established.
- The fifth factor is the reimbursement system in health care, which also plays a role. The reimbursement system is mainly focused on the care and treatment provided, and much less on (continuous) communication with the patient, in which care and treatment are geared to thinking from the perspective of patient needs and client needs.
- The last factor that influences the quality of care is that the health care system has a limited availability of resources. This can result in an increased demand on these limited resources. This can increase the pressure on healthcare professionals to make good use of these limited resources, because of which the healthcare professional may feel under stress, which limits his healthcare profession and may be at the expense of the patient (WHO 2003).

Integrated care is diametrically opposed to specialized and differentiated care. Specialized and differentiated care entails the risk of fragmentation of care and lower quality of care. Fragmentation of care has a negative impact on patient satisfaction as well as patient outcomes.

The current health care system has a strong focus on health problems and the biopsychosocial element is lost sight of. Integrated care is about integrating, connecting the care for patients at micro, meso, and macro levels. On a micro-level, it can be about integrating clinical care. At the meso-level, it can be about professional and organizational integration. And at the macro-level, about integrating systems (Goodwin 2013; Valentijn et al. 2013).

Integrated care can be made transparent based on a conceptual model, in which the care is divided at micro-level, meso-level, and macro-level (Valentijn et al. 2013):

– At the micro-level, it is about a coherent process of providing care to an individual patient, the clinical integration. Clinical integration is about coordinating care between professionals, and across institutional and sectoral boundaries.

Clinical integration means that you start from the patient situation with the aim of improving the patient's well-being and (as much as possible) promoting health.

Professionals must focus on patient needs from the patient's perspective. The care and treatment process are developed in co-creation with the patient, which means that form and content are given to the care process together with the patient. From the role of nursing professionals, we call this the co-creation of the care process. In this care process there is a shared responsibility between patient and care professional. The starting point here is the needs of the patient, whereby the patient can coordinate his own care if this is possible for him and desired by him.

– At the meso-level, an integration of organizations should arise to improve the efficiency and quality of care.

This integration also concerns professional integration and is the partnership between different professional groups in an organization and between different organizations.

This integration should provide a continuous, cohesive, and coordinated continuum of care appropriate to specific patient groups. Benefits are that care is more continuous, more interconnected, and better coordinated. It can be problematic that responsibility is shared, and decisions must be taken jointly by professionals.

– At the macro-level, the patient and his patient needs are placed at the center of the health care system. Subsequently, partnerships should be created between organizations to improve the efficiency and quality of care. A care continuum should be created, in which the patient or client is the focus of care.

Integrated, coherent care and good information transfer between (virtual) teams aims to eliminate the duplication of information and (diagnostic) tests (Davis et al. 2005).

Integrated care (or integrative medicine) combines approaches from both regular and alternative, complementary health care. Integral care provides care that is patient-centered, focused on healing and recovery with an emphasis on the (therapeutic) relationship, using approaches from both mainstream and complementary health care. According to Maizes and colleagues, complementary care requires a team approach, based on the biopsychosocial needs of the patient (Maizes et al. 2009).

There is medical dominance in healthcare. In both general and mental health care, the focus is on a medically oriented way of thinking. In this medical way of thinking, attention and actions are strongly aimed at solving (health) problems. The starting point is the disease, what knowledge of that disease do we have? And from there, what is the best way to deal with the disease? For example, knowledge focuses on taking antihypertensive medicines for a patient with high blood pressure. The best way to manage high blood pressure is for the patient to be prescribed antihypertensive drugs.

Within nursing care, the emphasis should be on care domination. The emphasis should then be on care-oriented thinking in both general and mental health care. In care-oriented thinking, the focus is much less on solution-oriented thinking. Nursing care should be about tailoring care to the needs of the patient. Care-oriented thinking is therefore less solution-oriented compared to medical thinking. However, this does not mean that nurses do not work towards "solving" the disease. It does mean that the patient's "disease" is placed in the context of providing good care. The nurse constantly looks at the patient's needs beyond the scope—of the patient's or client's physical or mental problem.

21.5 Conclusion

- Integrated care is a simple idea that involves combining different healthcare parts to form a whole that optimizes care and treatment.
- Integrated healthcare systems can enhance accessibility, quality, and continuity of healthcare services, making it easier to tailor care to individual patients. A lack of time and resources, the reimbursement system, and inadequate communication and information sharing between healthcare facilities can negatively impact patient outcomes.
- Integrative care is diametrically opposed to specialized and differentiated care, which can cause fragmentation of care and lower the quality of care. The integrative approach can be made transparent by dividing care at the micro, meso, and macro levels, where each level has its own benefits and challenges.
- Integrative care is not just about combining mainstream and complementary healthcare approaches, but it is also about a team approach, putting the patient's needs and preferences at the center of care.
- Overall, integrated care aims to eliminate the duplication of information and diagnostic tests while improving patient outcomes, satisfaction, and well-being.

- Integrated care is an approach that emphasizes coordinated care to improve the quality of patient care. It aims to address patient needs on a micro, meso, and macro levels, by improving communication and collaboration between healthcare professionals and organizations.
- Integrated care provides patient-centered, cohesive, and coordinated care.
- As healthcare resources become increasingly limited, integrated care can serve as a promising approach to provide the best possible care to patients.

Box 21.1 Mind-Map

Create a mind map on the position of the patient or client in an integrated care context.

Point out what the positive factors are for patient and clients.

Also indicate which negative factors there may be for the patient of clients.

Use: positive factors as: Tailored care and treatment; better coordination of care; improved health outcomes; patient-centered care; higher patient and family satisfaction; better relationship between patient, family, and healthcare professional; an holistic approach.

Use also negative factors for patient: Lack of communication between healthcare professionals; limited access to specialized care; fragmented care; poor coordination between health systems; lack of integration in information systems; and insufficient resources for integrated care.

Box 21.2 Mind-Map Nursing in the Context of Integrated Care

Create a mind map on the nurse in the context of integrated care.

Point out the positive factors for care professionals.

Point out the negative factors associated with this approach to providing care.

Additionally, identify three important factors that you think are crucial for a care professional in this context.

Use: Positive factors for a care professional in the context of integrated care include improved patient outcomes, greater job satisfaction through collaborative work with other healthcare professionals, and the ability to provide more holistic care tailored to the patient's needs. With integrated care, care professionals can enhance their knowledge and skills in different areas of care, which may lead to professional development opportunities.

Negative factors for care professionals may include the need for additional training to adapt to a collaborative work environment, time constraints when working with multiple care providers, and potential role conflicts between care providers.

Use important factors as effective communication and collaboration with other healthcare professionals, patient-centered care, focus on continuous professional development, providing high-quality, coordinated care that meets the needs of their patients while also ensuring their own job satisfaction and growth.

Box 21.3 Mind-Map Integrated Care, Benefit for Patients and Clients
Create a mind-map on integrated care and accessibility, quality, and continuity of services.

Explore how integrated care can benefit patients, healthcare professionals, and healthcare facilities, and the challenges that must be addressed to achieve integrated care.

Box 21.4 Mind-Map Advantages of Integrated Care
Create a mind-map on advantages of integrated care over specialized and differentiated care.

Explore the drawbacks of specialized and differentiated care and how integrated care can overcome these challenges.

Nursing and Intraprofessional and Interprofessional Cooperation

22

22.1 Topic List: Interprofessional Cooperation

1. Importance of effective interprofessional teams in healthcare: Cooperation, synergy, and patient-centered care.
2. Role of informed and active patients in collaborative care: Benefits of patient involvement in care and treatment.
3. Integrated care: Intraprofessional and interprofessional cooperation for improved patient outcomes.
4. Communication in collaborative care: Real-time contact and indirect communication methods.
5. Clinical reasoning and decision-making in collaborative care: Communication of facts and care-related recommendations.
6. Link between miscommunication and adverse patient outcomes: The impact of communication styles and differences between professional groups.
7. Clash of cultures between medical and non-medical professional groups: Challenges in providing integrated care and treatment.
8. Impact of communication styles on patient story presentation: Differences between nursing professionals and clinicians.
9. Factors influencing interprofessional communication: Lack of trust, experience, complexity of healthcare, and lack of structure.
10. Opportunities to improve interprofessional communication: Interprofessional tools and methods.
11. Best practices for optimizing interprofessional cooperation and overcoming communication problems in collaborative care.

B. Sassen, *Improving Person-Centered Innovation of Nursing Care*, https://doi.org/10.1007/978-3-031-35048-1_22

22.2   Introduction

The Collaborative Care model emphasizes the importance of effective teamwork between healthcare professionals and patients to achieve patient-centered, high-quality care. The model requires multidisciplinary teams of proactive care providers who work together to integrate prevention and cure into care and treatment. However, effective interprofessional collaboration depends on communication styles, professional socialization, and structural hierarchy, which can result in miscommunication and adverse patient outcomes. Therefore, it is crucial to understand these factors to enhance interprofessional communication and provide effective care.

Valentijn et al. (2013) highlighted the clash of cultures between medical and non-medical professional groups, which has made it difficult to integrate care and treatment. This dissonance between different professional perspectives can lead to ineffective communication between professionals, which can result in misdiagnoses, medication errors, treatment delays, and patient injury. Foronda et al. (2019) further noted that the communication style of nurses differs from that of physicians, leading to a difference in how the patient story is presented, with both professional groups communicating from their own frame and narrative structure. Despite the importance of effective interprofessional communication, many factors can negatively influence it, such as a lack of trust, experience, complexity of healthcare, concentrated attention-demanding activities, lack of structure, and lack of standardization of work (Foronda et al. 2016).

22.3   Topics

This chapter focuses on the Collaborative Care model, which emphasizes creating a positive and productive interaction between patients and healthcare professionals through effective interprofessional teamwork. The chapter discusses the importance of patient-centered care and the role of communication in achieving integrated care. It also highlights the benefits of collaborative care in managing major depressive disorders and improving patient outcomes.

The passage delves into the challenges of interprofessional communication, including differences in communication styles and the clash of cultures between medical and non-medical professional groups. Factors that negatively influence interprofessional communication are also discussed, along with opportunities to improve it, including interprofessional tools like the SBAR method.

Overall, the chapter emphasizes the importance of effective teamwork and communication in providing high-quality patient care.

22.4 Effective Working Together

The Collaborative Care model is about creating a positive, productive interaction between patients and the team of healthcare professionals. Effective teams are teams in which cooperation arises, where the whole is greater than the sum of its parts. And an effective team is a team in which professionals of all backgrounds work together to achieve results of care that any single professional could not achieve alone (Atlantis et al. 2014). In such an interprofessional team, synergy arises when work is targeted, people actively listen to each other, the professionals feel involved and flexible, and show commitment to the jointly made decisions. Interprofessional teams are essential for patient-centered, high-quality care.

The interaction can best take shape when patients or clients are informed and take an active, directing position in the communication with healthcare providers. Healthcare providers should work together in a multidisciplinary team, with each team member taking a proactive position. An informed and active patient in a mutually productive interaction with a multidisciplinary team of proactive care providers will result in integrated care, in which prevention and cure are integrated into care and treatment (Fig. 22.1; Wagner et al. 1996; Glasgow et al. 2003).

Integrated care requires cooperation within the same professional group (intraprofessional cooperation) and cooperation between different professional groups (interprofessional cooperation). The communication flows take place in real time, in direct contact between people. This happens during consultation moments, rounds, preliminary discussions, transfer or other direct personal contact. In addition to this real-time contact, indirect communication takes place via electronic patient records, medication orders, written notes, and e-mail contact (Foronda et al. 2019).

Developed from the Chronic Care model collaborative care improves the management of people with major depressive disorders. A meta-analysis shows that collaborative care has a positive effect on a return to work and on productivity. The Collaborative Care model provides patients with a supportive network, encouraging them to take a more active role in their own care (Thota et al. 2012).

For effective interprofessional collaboration, it is important for nursing professionals to communicate the facts with skill and to indicate the clinical problem, with targeted (care-related) recommendations. Based on clinical reasoning, clinical decision-making can thus be reached.

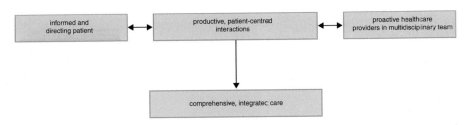

Fig. 22.1 Integrated care ((naar: (Wagner et al. 1996; Glasgow et al. 2003) beeldrechten: [rechten bij auteur] bestand)

A review describes that there is a link between miscommunication between professionals and adverse patient outcomes (The Joint Commission 2015, in: Foronda, MacWilliams and McArthur 2016) and that interprofessional communication depends on the different communication styles between professional groups (Foronda et al. 2016). These differences in communication styles have to do with education, structural hierarchy, and professional socialization.

Valentijn et al. (2013) speak of the clash of cultures between medical and non-medical professional groups in that respect. That is one reason why providing integrated care and treatment is difficult. Foronda et al. (2019) refer to this as a dissonance between the holistic perspective of nurses, which is complex, while physicians adopt a more objective perspective (Foronda et al. 2016). Ineffective communication between professionals can lead to misdiagnoses, medication errors, treatment delays, and patient injury.

The communication style of nurses has evolved from their education and professional socialization, as a "this is how we do it" in a rather descriptive way of communicating. The communication style of doctors also originated from training and professional socialization, as a rather compact, concise way of communicating. As a result, there is a difference in how the patient story is presented: both professional groups do this from their own frame and narrative structure (Foronda et al. 2019).

Both communication styles are perceived differently by the other profession. Nursing professionals experience the compact, concise way of describing a patient story as having little regard for the patient's individuality, as not-attention, as unwillingness to discuss the goals. This gives nursing professionals the feeling that they must provide a list of signs and symptoms. Clinicians perceive the descriptive way of presenting a patient story as less organized, illogical, unprepared to discuss the patient, as irrelevant information and as a delaying element to get to the point (Foronda et al. 2016).

Factors that negatively influence interprofessional communication are a lack of trust, lack of experience, the complexity of healthcare, the concentrated attention-demanding activities of healthcare, lack of structure and lack of standardization of work (Foronda et al. 2016). Opportunities to improve interprofessional communication are shown in Fig. 22.2.

Interprofessional tools are available to optimize interprofessional cooperation and overcome communication problems. For example, the SBAR (Situation Background Assessment and Recommendation) appears to reduce the probability of errors (Table 22.1). This method is useful in nearly all medical situations that may arise in hospitals, and uses a brief introduction and telling what is wrong with the patient or client; list of relevant points from the patient's history and course of illness; summarizing findings and stating conclusion; and make a treatment proposal and indicate what is required for this.

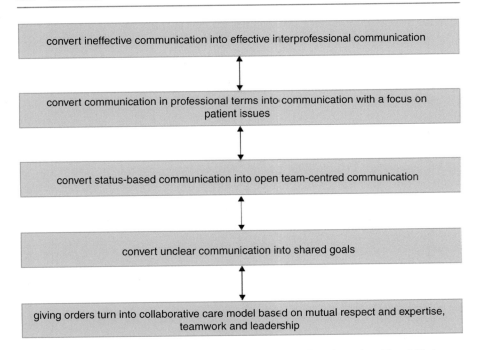

Fig. 22.2 Improving the interprofessional communication. (Based on: Arnold and Underman Boggs 2020 beeldrechten: [rechten bij auteur] bestand)

Table 22.1 Situation background assessment recommendation

Situation	Give a brief introduction of the patient and tell your colleagues what is wrong with him or her
Background	List relevant points from the patient's history (including patient needs) and course of illness
Assessment	Give a summary of your findings and include a conclusion
Recommendation	Make a treatment proposal and indicate which healthcare professionals and which treatment(s) and medication/aids are required

22.5 Conclusion

- The Collaborative Care model emphasizes the importance of creating a positive, productive interaction between patients and healthcare professionals through interprofessional teamwork.
- Effective interprofessional teams are essential for providing patient-centered, high-quality care that integrates prevention and cure.
- Communication is key to effective collaboration, and both real-time and indirect communication channels should be utilized.
- The Collaborative Care model has shown positive results in managing disorders, and interprofessional tools can help optimize communication and reduce errors.

- However, interprofessional communication can be hindered by differences in communication styles between professional groups, lack of trust, experience, structure, and standardization of work. By addressing these challenges, healthcare professionals can provide integrated care that meets patients' needs and expectations. Opportunities to improve interprofessional communication include using standardized tools and creating a culture of mutual respect and trust.
- Effective communication between medical professionals is crucial for providing safe and high-quality patient care. However, differences in communication styles and lack of trust and experience can negatively impact interprofessional communication, leading to errors and patient harm. Therefore, it is essential to address these challenges and promote effective interprofessional communication through training, standardization of work processes, and creating a culture of mutual respect and understanding between medical professionals.

Box 22.1 Mind-Map Clashing of Cultures
Make a mind-map on the clashing of cultures versus intra- and interprofessional collaboration.
   When examining the conflicts that can arise from cultural differences and the need for collaboration among healthcare professionals within and across fields:
   What opportunities exist for growth and cooperation.
   What challenges must be overcome and how?

Box 22.2 Mind-Map Importance of Interprofessional Teamwork
Create a mind-map on the importance of effective interprofessional teamwork for patient-centered, high-quality care.
   Point out the benefits of collaborative care for managing major disorders, make this specific from the patient perspective.

Box 22.3 Mind-Map Challenges of Interprofessional Communication
Create a mind-map on the challenges of interprofessional communication and strategies to improve it.
   Point out factors that negatively influence interprofessional communication and explore strategies to improve interprofessional communication.

Box 22.4 Mind-Map Effective Interprofessional Collaboration
Create a mind-map on the role of nurses in effective interprofessional collaboration.

Point out your own role in effective interprofessional collaboration.

Use interprofessional collaboration and communication; holistic perspective clash, and communication styles in nursing and how these are perceived.

Nursing and Shared Governance and Professional Governance

23

23.1 Topic List

1. Definition and principles of shared governance as an organizational strategy that empowers nursing professionals in decision-making and care provision.
2. Benefits of shared governance, including increased nurse and patient satisfaction, improved nursing care, and better patient outcomes.
3. Importance of communication and collaboration among team members in shared governance, including barriers to effective team communication.
4. Holacracy model and its emphasis on the importance of each team member's opinion in patient-centered care.
5. Role of nursing leadership in implementing shared governance and creating a patient-centered culture.
6. Balancing patient values and organizational values in nursing care provision and the impact of organizational support on patient-centered care.
7. Decentralized decision-making and the involvement of healthcare professionals in policy development and implementation.
8. Influence of shared governance on job satisfaction, burnout, performance, and retention of nursing professionals.
9. Successful implementation of shared governance, such as Magnet hospitals, and the need for formal structures and processes to support nurse involvement in decision-making.
10. Challenges and limitations of implementing shared governance in healthcare organizations.
11. Importance of shared governance as a key component in achieving patient-centered care and improving nursing practice.

© The Author(s), under exclusive license to Springer Nature
Switzerland AG 2023
B. Sassen, *Improving Person-Centered Innovation of Nursing Care*,
https://doi.org/10.1007/978-3-031-35048-1_23

23.2   Introduction

Providing patient-centered care requires changes at both the individual healthcare professional and organizational levels. Shared governance, a non-hierarchical decision-making model, is an effective organizational strategy that allows nursing professionals to take ownership of nursing care and provide input in professional care provision. Shared governance increases nurse involvement, autonomy, job satisfaction, and decision-making power, which has a positive impact on patient care and safety. The concept of shared governance has benefits for nursing practice.

23.3   Topics

The chapter discusses the concept of shared governance, which is an organizational strategy that enables nursing professionals to take ownership of nursing care, be autonomous, and provide input in professional care provision. Shared governance is a key component in improving nursing care, as it increases both patient and nurse satisfaction.

Shared governance requires changes at both the individual healthcare professional and organizational levels of healthcare institutions. It discusses that nursing professionals should actively participate in consultations in places where institutional policy is determined, influencing decisions that affect direct patient care at the micro, meso, and macro levels.

Shared governance helps ensure that the professionals who provide direct care become part of decision-making processes, and it is about creating organizational structures that give nursing staff more influence over their own work, offering more autonomy to make decisions. Shared governance involves non-hierarchical decision-making. Magnet hospitals are proof that high levels of nurse involvement in hospital decision-making is not a utopia. Shared governance is a powerful tool to improve the job satisfaction of professionals, the quality of the care provided, and patient safety, as well as to retain professionals in the organization.

23.4   Shared Professional Governance

For patient-centered care to be successful, this requires changes at both the level of individual healthcare professionals and at the organizational level of healthcare institutions. In this respect, it is desirable that the style of leadership is not based on control and management, but on joint management, we call this shared governance (Hobbs 2009, in: Morgan and Yoder 2012).

Shared governance increases the involvement of nursing professionals in care by allowing them to think along with the entire healthcare organization and give them decision-making power (Kutney-Lee et al. 2016). Shared governance is therefore an organizational strategy that enables nurses to take ownership of nursing care, to be autonomous, and to be able to provide input in professional care provision (Yoder-Wisse 2019).

Shared governance is a key component in improving nursing care (Valentijn et al. 2013). It is based on the principles of partnership, equality, taking responsibility and ownership (Porter-O'Grady 2003). It is the way to empower nurses to manage nursing practice (Yoder-Wisse 2019). Shared governance increases both patient and nurse satisfaction (Kutney-Lee et al. 2016).

Working together to reach joint decisions and working together in the coordination of care requires commitment at the right time, but also to hold on and let go at the right time (Arnold and Underman Boggs 2020). According to the Holacracy model, the opinion of each team member is important, and the starting point is:

No one wins unless everyone wins.

Based on patient needs, the goals of care and treatment are leading in the communication between team members and all communication is focused on these patient needs (Arnold and Underman Boggs 2020).

Giving the nursing profession the decision-making power, especially regarding direct patient care, increases the involvement of nurses in the organization (Kutney-Lee et al. 2016). Nurses should actively participate in consultations in places where institutional policy is determined, thus influencing the decisions that affect direct patient care at the micro-level, but also at the meso and macro levels.

According to Yoder-Wisse (2019), when we talk about shared governance, it is essentially about shared decision-making. Shared governance offers professionals an organizational structure in which it is possible to make decisions at a decentralized level. This enables nurses to identify problems related to patient-centered care, develop solutions, and test and implement healthcare innovations (Yoder-Wisse 2019). Implementing an organizational model according to the principles of shared governance requires nursing leadership (Yoder-Wisse 2019).

The core idea of shared governance is to put the relationship at the center of care planning, as opposed to the task at the center. Putting the relationship at the center of shared governance fits in seamlessly with putting the relationship at the center of patient-centered care. Nurses always balance between patient values and organizational values in the provision of care (Morgan and Yoder 2012). A lack of support from the organization to create and maintain a patient-centered culture prevents nurses from providing patient-centered care (Morgan and Yoder 2012).

Barriers to making team communication more effective are (TeamSTEPPS 2017, in: Arnold and Underman Boggs 2020):

- not sharing information between team members;
- a hierarchical structure in the team that makes the opinion of one person more important than the opinion of the other;
- variation in communication styles or vocabulary between professional groups;
- lack of flexibility;
- feeling attacked;
- existence of conflicts.

Shared governance helps ensure that the professionals who provide direct care become part of decision-making processes. Shared governance is, in fact, shared decision-making between line and staff management. Previously, it was decided from above how healthcare professionals should carry out their work, now they are involved in making decisions themselves. Shared governance is therefore about decentralized decision-making and being present at important crossroads in the organization where policies that affect patient care are determined. If this influence of healthcare professionals is not there, and decisions are made by managers outside of patient care, this will have undesirable effects. Where decisions are made that affect direct patient care or professional practice, it is important that healthcare professionals also have an influence on this. They must be able to co-decide on the policies and procedures that they must implement themselves in practice. They must be heard when it comes to this and help determine which changes must be implemented "on the shop floor."

Direct involvement of professionals in the policy pursued increases the job satisfaction of professionals and reduces the chances of burnout. The performance of professionals in direct patient care is improving, the quality of the care provided is increasing and patient safety is also optimized. Finally, this also has a positive influence on the retention of professionals for the organization because professionals are less inclined to leave (Kutney-Lee et al. 2016).

Shared governance is about creating organizational structures that give nursing staff more influence over their own work, offering more autonomy to make decisions. Shared governance involves non-hierarchical decision-making. A good example of this non-hierarchical decision-making and shared governance has been implemented in Magnet hospitals (Kutney-Lee et al. 2016). The features of the Magnet principle have a positive effect on patient care and a positive effect on the working environment (Kutney-Lee et al. 2016). To obtain a Magnet status as a hospital, a system of quality improvement must be met. This quality system must demonstrate that nurses have a clear role in institutional policy and decision-making (Kutney-Lee et al. 2016).

Magnet hospitals are proof that high levels of nurse involvement in hospital decision-making is not a utopia. However, formal structures and processes must be implemented that allow for the influence of nurses (Kutney-Lee et al. 2016). In organizations where professional autonomy is stimulated, this leads to more job satisfaction, higher productivity, and less turnover among professionals (Fisher et al. 2016).

There is a development from shared governance to professional governance. At its core, professional governance is about taking responsibility, making a professional commitment, reciprocal relationships, and effective decision-making (Clavelle et al. 2016).

To provide safe, high-quality care, there should be a collaborative, patient-centered care model, where all team members are valued for the role they play. This means that all team members work together in their pursuit of the maximum achievable health outcomes for each patient. This they do by (Arnold and Underman Boggs 2020):

- working on a common goal;
- communicating openly and securely;
- treating all team members with respect;
- ensuring joint decision-making in the team;
- clearing roles within the team;
- clear communication, both verbal and written.

23.5 Conclusion

- The concept of shared governance is an organizational strategy to empower nursing professionals to take ownership of nursing care, be autonomous, and provide input in professional care provision.
- Shared governance enables nurses to make decisions at a decentralized level and identify problems related to patient-centered care, develop solutions, and test and implement healthcare innovations.
- In shared governance, key is the importance of shared decision-making, nurse involvement in policymaking, and creating organizational structures that give nursing staff more influence over their own work. Magnet hospitals are based on non-hierarchical decision-making and shared governance, which has a positive effect on patient care and the working environment.
- Shared governance is an organizational strategy that empowers nurses to take ownership of their nursing practice and provide input in decision-making processes. It is based on the principles of partnership, equality, taking responsibility, and ownership and enables nurses to identify problems related to patient-centered care and develop solutions.
- Shared governance increases nurse involvement, autonomy, job satisfaction, and decision-making power, which ultimately leads to improved patient care and safety.
- Organizations must implement formal structures and processes that allow for the influence of nurses to achieve high levels of nurse involvement and autonomy. Shared governance is a key component in improving nursing care and should be a priority for healthcare institutions that strive to provide patient-centered care.

Box 23.1 Mind-Map to Support Nursing Involvement in Decision-Making
Create a mind-map. The role of Magnet hospitals as examples of successful implementation of shared governance and the need for formal structures and processes to support nursing involvement in decision-making.

Indicate how shared governance can be achieved: where in the organization should nursing professionals "sit" to optimize patient care or to create and guarantee optimal patient care?

Link the places in the organization to themes on which nurses could exert influence.

For example: at the team level, nurses can influence…; at the departmental level, nurses can influence…; etc.

Background: To achieve shared governance in healthcare organizations, it is important to determine where nursing professionals should be positioned to optimize patient care and ensure its quality. This involves linking the places in the organization to the themes on which nurses can exert influence. For instance, at the team level, nurses can influence the coordination of patient care and communication with patients and their families. At the departmental level, they can influence policies and procedures related to nursing care and patient safety. In addition, nurses can have an impact on resource allocation and budget decisions at the organizational level. By positioning nursing professionals strategically throughout the organization and giving them the authority to influence these key areas, shared governance can be achieved, resulting in improved patient outcomes and higher job satisfaction for nurses.

Box 23.2 Mind-Map Importance of Shared Governance
Create a mind-map on the importance of shared governance in promoting patient-centered care and improving nursing practice.

Point out the benefits of shared governance for nursing professionals.

Point out why shared decision-making and non-hierarchical decision-making structures improve job satisfaction and reduce burnout among healthcare professionals.

Nursing and Evidence-Based Practice   24

24.1   Topic List for Change and Innovation Based on Evidence-Based Practice in Nursing

1. Importance of evidence-based practice in nursing: foundation of nursing care, moving away from traditional approaches based on habit or consensus.
2. Responsibility of nurses in critically analyzing the best available evidence from scientific literature and integrating it into nursing diagnoses and interventions for achieving favorable patient outcomes.
3. Positive impact of evidence-based practice on improving the targeting and effectiveness of care and treatment in healthcare settings.
4. Challenge of integrating scientific insights with patient needs to provide person-centered care, focusing on the individual needs and preferences of patients while considering evidence-based practices.
5. Importance of recognizing the limits of nursing expertise and consulting with other healthcare professionals, diving into the literature, and referring to appropriate resources to provide evidence-based care.
6. Avoiding unnecessary interventions that lack evidence-based rationale, such as unnecessary procedures or medications.
7. Limitations of clinical guidelines: Exploring the limitations of clinical guidelines and the need to consider the patient perspective to improve patient well-being, rather than solely relying on guidelines.
8. Reassurance based on expertise: Emphasizing the importance of providing reassurance to patients based on evidence-based expertise.
9. Building a solid foundation for nursing care: Highlighting how evidence-based practice serves as the foundation for nursing care, enabling nursing professionals to provide high-quality care based on the best available evidence.

© The Author(s), under exclusive license to Springer Nature
Switzerland AG 2023
B. Sassen, *Improving Person-Centered Innovation of Nursing Care*,
https://doi.org/10.1007/978-3-031-35048-1_24

24.2   Introduction

Evidence-based practice has become a cornerstone of modern healthcare, and it is essential that nursing professionals systematically analyze the best available evidence from scientific literature to achieve favorable patient outcomes. This approach has significantly improved the targeting and effectiveness of care by moving away from outdated practices based on tradition or consensus and toward a more patient-centered approach.

The challenge now is to use scientific insights as a starting point and to consider patient needs from there, ensuring that patient outcomes are meaningful and valuable. This chapter will explore the benefits and challenges of evidence-based practice in nursing care and how it can be integrated with patient-centered care.

Benefits of using scientific evidence are to improve the targeting and effectiveness of care and treatment, but it emphasizes the need to prioritize patient needs in decision-making. It is important to consult others and the literature when necessary, avoiding unnecessary actions, and providing reassurance based on expertise. Clinical guidelines also call for a focus on the patient perspective to improve overall patient well-being.

24.3   Topics

This chapter discusses the importance of evidence-based practice in nursing care and how it has improved the targeting and effectiveness of care. This chapter emphasizes the need to start from patient needs and enter into a conversation with the patient about what evidence-based care and treatment best fits their needs. The challenge is discussed how to use scientific insights as a starting point while also looking at patient needs from a person-centered or patient-centered perspective. The passage highlights the importance of providing care based on evidence, not tradition or consensus-based practices, and consulting others outside one's immediate professional group to ensure the best care for patients. Limitations of clinical guidelines are discussed, next to the importance of emphasizing a patient-centered focus to improve patient well-being.

24.4   Evidence-Based Person-Centered Care

Change and innovation in health care should have its origins in evidence-based practice. Nurses should be focused on systematically analyzing best available evidence from the scientific literature, linked to nursing diagnoses, and its relationship to implementation of nursing interventions aimed at achieving favorable patient outcomes. Targeted innovations should be deployed as much as possible based on the best available evidence. Nursing professionals would thus work to build a solid foundation for nursing care (Yoder-Wisse 2019).

The development that care and treatment should stem from the best available evidence has done a lot of good for healthcare. Because we now have a better understanding of the underlying, scientific evidence for nursing practice, the targeting and effectiveness of care has undoubtedly increased. Whereas in the past nurses and other health care providers were more often providing care and treatment based on "that's just the way we do it," we have now mostly meaningfully moved away from that.

The transition to care and treatment based on evidence-based practice has undoubtedly improved care. The descriptions in guidelines and protocols, insofar as they are not only consensus-based but especially evidence-based, have given a positive boost to care and treatment. Now we are at the point where we should start from patient needs, start from the specific patient or client situation, the person as a holistic unit. And from here (from these patient needs) enter conversation with the patient about what evidence-based care and treatment (from your professional knowledge and insight) best fits his or her needs.

The challenge is to use scientific insights as a starting point and to look at patient needs from there. Scientific insights are the underpinning of one's nursing actions. Person-centered or patient-centered care with its focus on the individual needs of patients and clients seems to be at odds with evidence-based practice, which focuses on needs of groups and populations. However, good patient outcome should be defined in terms of what is important, meaningful and valuable to the individual patient. So based on what has been proven effective in research, look at how this can fit the needs of the individual patient. A patient outcome is only a good outcome if it fits the patient or client (Epstein and Street Jr. 2011). As a nurse, you need to think not only from the care and treatment offerings, but from the care needs and desires of the individual patient or client.

Nursing is providing care for which there is evidence—not because we "just do it that way." Knowing your own professional boundaries, and consulting others outside your immediate professional group, diving into the literature or referring if this becomes (further) outside your area of expertise, is part of this. Not doing unnecessary things that have been shown by literature search to have no rationale for this action, not prescribing medication if it can be done more simply. Patients ask for reassurance from expertise. Reassurance then means reassurance based on expertise, not false reassurance.

The limitations of clinical guidelines are increasingly apparent. Clinical integration requires a focus on the patient perspective to improve patient well-being, not just a focus on the guideline (Valentijn et al. 2013).

24.5 Conclusion

- The transition to evidence-based practice in healthcare has undoubtedly improved patient outcomes and the effectiveness of care. However, it is important to remember that patient-centered care is essential to providing the best possible care to individuals.

- Nursing professionals should use scientific evidence as a starting point and consider patient needs from there, ensuring that patient outcomes are meaningful and valuable. By doing so, healthcare providers can build a solid foundation for nursing care and promote innovation and change that will ultimately benefit patients.
- The limitations of clinical guidelines are increasingly apparent, and nursing professionals must focus on the patient perspective to improve patient well-being, not just the guideline.
- By combining evidence-based practice with patient-centered care, nursing professionals can continue to provide high-quality care that meets the needs of individual patients and clients.

Box 24.1 Mind-Map 1 Importance of Evidence-Based Practice
Make a mind-map on the importance of evidence-based practice for nursing professional and patients and clients.
   Point out the changes that evidence-based practice has brought for you as a nurse, state the benefits on the left side.
   Point out the benefits and side effects for patient and clients on the right side.
   Put arrows between similar factors.
   Circle the 3 most important factors as seen from your own perspective.

Box 24.2 Mind-Map 2 Relationship Between Evidence-Based Practice, Patient-Centered Care, and Innovation in Healthcare
Create a mind-map illustrating the relationship between evidence-based practice, patient-centered care, and innovation in healthcare.
   Instructions:

1. Start with a central concept, Healthcare Improvement.
2. Draw three branches representing Evidence-Based Practice, Patient-Centered Care, and Innovation.
3. Under the Evidence-Based Practice branch, include sub-branches like Systematic Analysis, Best Available Evidence, etc.
4. Under the Patient-Centered Care branch, include sub-branches for Patient Needs, Individual Care, and Patient Outcome.
5. Under the Innovation branch, include sub-branches for Targeted Innovations, Best Available Evidence, and Patient Well-being.
6. Connect the sub-branches to show the interdependence and relationship between evidence-based practice, patient-centered care, and innovation.
7. Add additional details or notes to the branches and sub-branches as needed to further develop the relationships and concepts.

Nursing and Quality of Care   25

25.1 Topic List on the Importance of Quality of Care

1. Quality of Life and Its Relationship with Health: How quality of care impacts patients' overall quality of life and well-being, and how health outcomes are closely related to the quality of care received
2. Recognizing the importance of autonomy in patients' decision-making and care preferences, and how respecting patient autonomy contributes to the quality of care provided.
3. The Impact of Illness Experience on Health Assessment and Quality of Life: Considering the unique experiences and perspectives of patients in assessing their health and quality of life, and how this impacts the quality of care provided.
4. Patient- or Person-Centered Care as an Essential Component of Quality of Care: The importance of placing the patient or person at the center of care, and how this approach enhances the quality of care provided.
5. Factors Influencing Patient Satisfaction and Its Positive Effects on Quality of Care.
6. Pillars for Improving Quality of Care: Patient Satisfaction, Performance Improvement, Regulatory Constraints, Clinical Effectiveness, and Patient Safety.
7. Patient-Centered, Relational Approach as the Key to Providing Quality Care: Highlighting the importance of building strong patient–provider relationships based on trust, empathy, and effective communication to ensure high-quality care.
8. Goals of Quality of Care: Interpersonal Relationships, Patient Involvement in Care, Coordination of Care, Integrated Care, Accessibility of Care, Information Systems, Patient-Centered Research, and Public Information about Health Care.
9. Understanding the various goals of quality of care and how they contribute to providing patient-centered care.

10. Recognizing that every interaction with the patient, from the first point of contact to the ongoing care, plays a crucial role in determining the overall quality of care provided.
11. Optimization of Access to Care and enhance the quality of care provided.
12. Exploring the challenges in providing cost-effective care while maintaining a patient-centered approach and finding solutions to overcome these challenges.
13. Recognizing the importance of patient experience in evaluating the quality of care received and the need to prioritize patient experience.
14. Factors Influencing Patient Experience in Health Care Settings, and their impact on the quality of care provided.
15. Relationship between Patient Experience and Perceived Quality of Care, patient experience contributes to improved quality of care and patient outcomes.
16. Impact of Patient Experience on Patient Safety, Clinical Effectiveness, and Health Outcomes, positive patient experience is linked to patient safety, clinical effectiveness, and improved health outcomes.
17. The critical role of nurses in improving patient experience and functional status.

25.2 Introduction

Quality of life is a multi-dimensional concept that encompasses various factors, including physical health and autonomy. The perception of quality of life changes when someone is ill, and it becomes essential to understand this change to provide appropriate care. Quality of care is critical in healthcare and involves policies and resources allocated to healthcare, as well as the welfare level of society. To determine good care, it is essential to adopt relational thinking and caregiving, which involve building relationships between patients and healthcare professionals, exchanging information, promoting self-management based on patient needs, and making decisions jointly. Nurses play a vital role in monitoring the quality of care and reflecting on their own actions to improve care continuously.

Patient-centered care is fundamental to quality of care, and it involves shared decision-making and improving patient satisfaction. A positive patient experience can improve perceived quality of care and patient safety, health outcomes, and medication and treatment adherence. Patient-centered care should be delivered in a manner that is accessible, coordinated, integrated, and involves patient involvement in care, research, and the availability of public information about healthcare. Providing quality care is more than just performing technical tasks, but it also involves building interpersonal relationships and engaging in patient-centered care delivery to promote patient autonomy and self-determination.

Quality of care is influenced by many factors, including the patient's needs and wants, cost considerations, market forces, and bureaucratic regulations. Healthcare professionals must focus on providing patient-centered, holistic, and individualized care that leads to improved health outcomes and quality of life. In this context, the relationship between the patient and healthcare professional is crucial, and professionals must involve patients in the care planning process. With the help of computer-based guidance and clinical information systems, healthcare professionals can improve the quality of care by accessing patient information, diagnostic tests, and decision-making support tools.

To optimize the quality of care, nursing professionals should use themselves as a tool to observe, assess, and improve the quality of care and establish a relationship with the patient to plan and coordinate care throughout the care process. The quality of care can be improved through good coordination of care and by emphasizing relational, collaborative care. Patient-reported outcome measures and patient-reported experience measures can also provide valuable feedback for healthcare professionals.

Quality of care is a crucial aspect of healthcare that involves patient-centered, holistic, and individualized care. It is heavily influenced by the purposefulness and focus of the organization providing care, and patients can also provide valuable feedback. Nursing professionals play a vital role in monitoring the quality of care and reflecting on their own actions to improve care continuously. Ultimately, providing good care requires healthcare professionals to think critically and integrate different dimensions into their practice to improve patient outcomes and quality of life.

25.3 Topics

The chapter explores the concept of quality of life and quality of care in healthcare settings. It discusses that quality of life should be considered beyond physical health and should include autonomy, emotional and relational aspects, and independent functioning. Similarly, quality of care should be patient-centered, with shared decision-making forming the foundation. Patient satisfaction, interpersonal relationships, coordination of care, accessibility of care, and adequate information systems are all critical elements of quality of care.

The chapter discusses that patient-centered care can be challenging to offer in a cost-effective manner and depends on the culture of the healthcare setting. However, nursing professionals who provide patient-centered care can contribute to the patient's functional capabilities and improve perceived quality of life and well-being. In this chapter the various aspects of healthcare, including market forces, professionalism, quality of care, nursing care, health gains, and the relationship between patients and healthcare professionals. The focus is on patient-centered care, which is holistic and individualized, and respects and empowers the patient. The increased use of technology in healthcare is highlighted and the need for healthcare professionals to involve patients and clients in the care planning process.

The chapter emphasizes the need for nursing professionals to use critical thinking and their own expertise to provide person-centered care to patients. The use of validated measurement tools, such as Patient Reported Outcome Measures (PROMs) and Patient Reported Experience Measures (PREMs), is also important to measure the quality of care. The text notes that good quality of care requires cohesion and continuity in care and emphasizes the importance of nursing professionals establishing a relationship with patients to plan and coordinate care throughout the care process. Peer review and quality promotion are also discussed as tools for improving the quality of care. The text highlights the importance of quality of life and quality of care in healthcare settings. It emphasizes the need for patient-centered care, the use of validated measurement tools, and the importance of nursing professionals establishing relationships with patients to plan and coordinate care. The ultimate goal is to improve patient outcomes and the quality of care provided.

25.4   Patient-Centered Quality of Care

Quality of life is often linked to health. But it also makes sense to link it to more than health and thus to draw quality of life broader. Quality of life can be given a broader perspective by linking it to autonomy. Seen from the perspective of autonomy, quality of care would mean that people's choice becomes more important. This involves questions such as: Can you arrange your life the way you want? Can you go to sleep, eat, or go outside if you want to?

When people are sick, this illness experience has an impact on their lives. Based on the illness experience, people assess their health differently, they adapt to being ill and assess their health and quality of life differently. As a result, they may rate the quality of life with illness as good (or even better) than the quality of life before their illness experience. It seems, as it were, that being ill has no impact on perceived quality of life, but of course this is not so. What matters is that people adapt to the new situation and view their lives in a different perspective. Understanding these adjustments and/or variations is important for adjusting care so that it is and remains focused on improving quality of life.

Quality of life consists of more aspects than mere health in the form of physical elements such as tightness and pain. It has emotional aspects, relational aspects, the degree of independent functioning, etc. The question, then, is quality of life sufficient for this patient? After all, it is the patient's own assessment. And it is not for the nurse or any other health care provider to make judgments about a patient's quality of life.

For quality of care, patient- or person-centered care is an essential component, where shared decision-making forms the foundation (Gill et al. 2019). A review shows that patient- and family-centered care is a key component to improve the quality of care (Yun and Choi 2019).

Patient satisfaction is strongly influenced by the quality of care provided. There are a number of factors that positively influence patient satisfaction, and thus quality of care. If the quality of care provided is high, it affects patient satisfaction with care, and this has positive effects on patient behavior, such as loyalty (Naidu 2009).

The focus for quality of care is on patient satisfaction, performance improvement, and regulatory constraints. These are the entry points for improving quality of care and are called the pillars of quality, along with clinical effectiveness and patient safety (McCarthy et al. 2016) (see Box 25.1).

Box 25.1 Pillars for Improving Quality of Care (McCarthy et al. 2016)
The pillars of quality of care described in the given conclusions are as follows:

1. Patient Satisfaction: This refers to the patient's perception of the care they receive and their overall satisfaction with it. It is important to consider patient satisfaction as a crucial aspect of quality care.
2. Performance Improvement: This involves continuously assessing and improving the quality of care provided to patients. This can be achieved by using quality management systems, guidelines, and protocols.
3. Regulatory Constraints: Quality care must adhere to regulatory constraints and guidelines. Healthcare providers need to be aware of and follow established rules and regulations.
4. Clinical Effectiveness: Quality care must be effective in achieving the desired outcomes. This involves using evidence-based practices and guidelines to provide appropriate care to patients.
5. Patient Safety: Patient safety is a critical aspect of quality care. Healthcare providers must ensure that patients are safe from harm and that the risk of adverse events is minimized.

Overall, providing quality care requires a patient-centered, relational approach that focuses on the individual needs and preferences of the patient and involves productive interactions between patients and healthcare providers. Continuous assessment and improvement of the quality of care can help to promote patient satisfaction, better outcomes, and a positive patient experience.

Quality of care, in addition to patient-centered care, has a number of goals (Davis et al. 2005). The interpersonal relationship between healthcare professionals among themselves and with care recipients is the most important measure for determining quality of care. In addition to this emphasis on interpersonal relationships (which is consistent with relational caregiving), quality of care is always about (Morgan and Yoder 2012):

– Patient involvement in care;
– Coordination of care;
– Integrated care by a team of professionals;
– The accessibility of care;
– Adequate information systems;
– Patient-centered research;
– The availability of public information about health care.

Providing quality care is more than performing a particular task technically well. Every interaction the patient has determines the quality of care and this means that care that is patient-centered improves the perceived quality of care (McCormack 2003).

While patient-centered care is an important component of quality of care, a gap exists between the care patients receive and the care patients should receive. Access to care would be optimized if appointment scheduling were made easier. This also means that appointments that are made fit well with patients' daily activities, there are shorter wait times, faster response times, and efficient use of patient time (Davis et al. 2005).

Patient-centered care is an important element of quality of care, but it remains a challenge to offer patient-centered care in a cost-effective manner (Bertakis and Azari 2011). For example, the culture in the setting affects a professional's ability to offer patient-centered care. This can both promote and hinder patient-centered care delivery and is determined by the people who lead and promote a certain vision and commitment. If they convey the importance of respectful care and the possibility of patient autonomy and self-determination, this is affirming for health care professionals (Fig. 25.1).

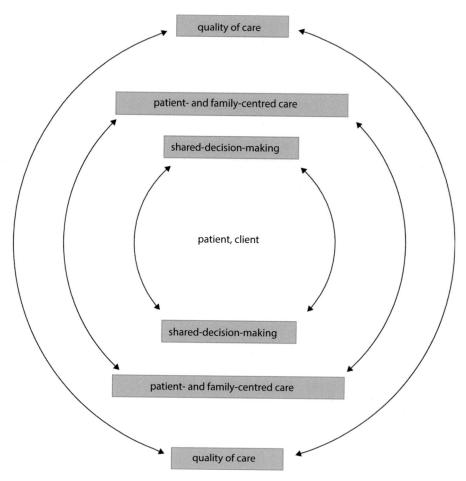

Fig. 25.1 The patient's relationship to quality of care

Patients gain experiences in contact with health care providers. These experiences significantly influence how they subsequently rate the contact or a series of encounters and interactions. The patient experience is based on the patient's feelings, assessment of the quality of care and treatment provided, and the perceived benefits they experience in doing so (Johnston and Kong 2011). If the patient experience is high, it also leads to a better perceived quality of care. A favorable patient experience has a positive relationship with patient safety, clinical effectiveness, health outcomes, utilization of health care services, and medication and treatment adherence (McCarthy et al. 2016).

Health outcomes are about the patient's functional status. Functional status is linked to the patient's roles at home and work, in society, their ADL activities, ability to communicate, and ability to participate in family, work, and social situations. Nurses who provide patient-centered care contribute to the patient's functional capabilities and thereby improve perceived quality of life and well-being.

The patient experience consists of rational aspects and functional aspects (Doyle et al. 2013). Rational aspects involve the interpersonal aspects of care, the patient's expectation that the professional has the patient's best interests at heart. In that regard, consider the patient's expectation that professionals have compassion for patients, are respectful, facilitate the patient to take care of their own health by providing empowerment, and include family and friends in the decision-making process. Functional aspects of care include patient expectations that health care services provide efficient and effective care, are hygienic and safe.

The effect of patient-centered communication on health outcomes will often not be immediately apparent. Therefore, it is important to pursue proximal outcomes (short-term goals). For example, that the patient feels understood that there is a bond of trust, that the patient is allowed to express their opinion, that the patient is motivated to change, and so on. The pursuit of these goals is desirable in any healthcare relationship, whether or not they are (directly) related to patient outcomes (Stewart et al. 2000).

Quality of care is also about the healthcare organization with its care processes, clinical information systems, decision-making processes, and the complex system around promoting patient self-management (Wagner et al. 1996). The health care system is focused on improving outcomes, both patient outcomes (such as well perceived quality of life) and care outcomes (such as good quality of care). The health care system is a part of the overall society, and this involves the (public health) policies and resources allocated to health care, among other things, as well as the welfare level of society. While health care today is mostly organized from institutional standards and routines, guidelines, and standardized procedures, it would make much more sense to organize it from patient needs and preferences (Suhonen et al. 2002). These should determine care.

The whole of society and healthcare system aims to achieve favorable patient outcomes at the intersection of productive interactions between the informed, active patient and the proactive team of healthcare providers.

Thinking from relational caregiving, determining quality of care is about what has gone well in care (Baart 2018). Relational thinking and relational caregiving also touch on quality of care and quality systems. Quality of care is then about the practice of caring, is about what is good. Quality of care is then about the right relationship to the fragility of life. All these factors determine good care, according to Baart (2018).

To assess care and see how care can be improved, the domains of patient-centered care can be used. When you think from these domains, health care facilities can improve and thus quality of care can improve (McCormack et al. 2011). This involves:

- Whether relationships are built between patients and health care professionals;
- Whether information is exchanged between patient and health care professionals;
- Whether healthcare professionals respond appropriately to patient stress and emotions;
- Whether healthcare professionals deal adequately with patient uncertainties;
- Whether decisions are taken jointly, and whether decision aids are used adequately in this process;
- Whether self-management is promoted based on patient needs.

Quality care requires quality awareness (Baart 2018). For quality care, the starting point is that care is provided relationally. Who can determine whether good quality care has been provided? According to the insights of relational caregiving, this is determined by those (patient and nurse) involved in the care. Those involved go to see for themselves whether good care was provided and then judge whether it was good quality care. The patient can judge whether good care has been provided.

Active and empowered patients can help improve care by pointing out where gaps in care exist. They can point out that they received incomplete information, that there was no shared decision-making, that care did not adequately meet their healthcare needs, that treatment was not perceived as appropriate, or that they need a second opinion.

If nurses continuously self-review and assess, quality awareness can emerge. If all nursing professionals are intradisciplinary focused on watching and assessing quality, quality awareness can emerge within the profession.

Monitoring the quality of care and making improvements based on it will promote patient satisfaction (Naidu 2009). To measure quality of care, outcomes of patient-centered care are important (Kogan et al. 2015).

Nurses look at the quality of care from their own point of view, and patients look at the quality of care from their position as patients. Nurses use guidelines, protocols, and standards, the premise being that working according to them leads to favorable patient outcomes and quality care. But quality care always requires a clear involvement of the individual patient in the care. While guidelines, protocols, and standards indicate how to proceed with certain disease states, it is important for nurses to always make this patient-centered. So, while the mostly evidence-based, but at least practice-based guidelines, protocols and standards reflect the agreements about the appropriate care for a particular disease state, nurses are also expected to always put themselves in the patient's shoes to determine what the appropriate care is for this particular patient.

Continually working on quality of care requires nursing professionals to reflect on their own actions and reflect with others on the care and treatment provided. This begins with analyzing and reflecting on the care they themselves have provided. The starting point is for nurses to analyze and reflect on their own care; elements of personal analysis and reflection may recur in a consultation, after which it is built upon to arrive at renewed insights or to confirm existing practices and actions.

Within health care, it is about results oriented work, effect measurements and market forces. Quality of care is measuring what the patient needs and what care the patient received. Quality of care means placing more and more value on patients' wants and needs, in which the cost aspect may play a role.

Freidson writes in his book Third Logic (2001):

Professionalism is a method of organizing work.

And:

In ideal-typical professionalism, specialized workers control their own work, [...] and practice influences the strength of professionalism.

International and national (health) policies influence the work of healthcare professionals. Even within the health care sector, professionals are increasingly confronted with market forces and bureaucratic regulations. Freidson (2001) says about this that the profession of healthcare professionals is weakening, this because under the guise of efficiency more and more is being asked and demanded of healthcare. About the position of healthcare professionals, he reports:

Their position is being seriously weakened in the name of competition and efficiency.

Healthcare professionals are increasingly caught between bureaucracy and market forces. This creates an ever-increasing division of labor, with tasks being "split up" for the purpose of providing efficient care. Because of this splitting up and specialization in subfields, it has become even more important to provide good care. For while specialization may lead to an improvement in efficient and effective care, in doing so, as a healthcare professional, you are more likely to become removed from unique, context-specific patient care. Freidson (2001) focuses on the independence of the professional and speaks of the superior value (transcendent value) of the professional. He sees this as an intrinsic value of professionals.

Nursing care should always focus on quality of life. Does the nursing care provided lead to an improvement or at least maintenance of the patient's quality of life? Within health care, we should always choose this path as much as possible: does care lead to (more) optimal quality of life for the patient? With care and treatment, there is now a strong focus on achieving favorable clinical outcomes. Treatment consists of choosing the most effective, evidence-based, treatment with the best prospects for the best outcomes. But as technical, specialized and differentiated treatments continue to increase, and especially as technology continues to improve, this makes health care increasingly sophisticated. This makes the question increasingly important, whether this also results in satisfaction giving quality of life.

Besides the fact that nursing care should focus on the quality of life perceived favorably by the patient, it is also about health gains. In addition to favorably perceived quality of life, does the care actually deliver health gains? Quality of life has a lot to do with shortening the duration of treatment. Patient treatment can be viewed as a process from health complaint, through procedures, referrals, and treatments to the end of treatment. The patient's perceived quality of life and ultimate health gain are strongly influenced by this process. These procedures, referrals, and treatments can be more favorable to the patient in two ways. Optimizing these components by allowing patient preferences to play a clear role in them within the entirety of relational, patient-centered care can improve patient well-being. Optimizing these parts of the process by improving effectiveness and efficiency in them can improve the patient's perceived quality of life and promote health care cost-effectiveness. Unnecessary procedures, referrals, and care and treatment are avoided.

The relationship between patient and healthcare professional can be key. Whether a nursing or medical intervention produces the intended result is often not clear in advance. Healthcare professionals used to enter an obligation of effort, whereas now the goal is mostly an obligation of result, with goal achievement and efficiency as important parameters. This limits professional space, but because professionals have control over their own work, professional space should also be filled with providing relational care to patients in their unique contextual situations. This means that healthcare professionals have specialized knowledge and skills through expertise, which can be tailored to the patient as they see fit. In doing so, the healthcare professional moves away from the norm of result-oriented professional action and the rather strictly defined frameworks within the provision of care.

For quality of care, it involves patient-centered care that is holistic and individualized, respectful, and empowering for the patient. If care meets these core elements of patient-centered care, it will lead to improved quality of care, greater satisfaction with care, and improved health outcomes (Fig. 25.2) (Morgan and Yoder 2012).

A systematic review shows that involving patients in the planning and implementation of care is complex. The experiences and satisfaction of patients and clients are factors that can influence changes in health care, but health care professionals are the ones who ultimately determine how much value is placed on them. Professionals will increasingly need to be able to demonstrate that they properly involve patients and clients in the care planning process, but they remain accountable for the professional decisions they make (Crawford et al. 2002).

The professional is (increasingly) supported by computer-based guidance and clinical information systems, such as electronic health records available everywhere. These clinical information systems can support and enable high-quality care. For example, through access to laboratory findings and diagnostic tests, as well as patient reminders, decision support tools, longitudinal understanding of risk factors, and utilization of health services (Davis et al. 2005). Increasingly, technology support consists of biomedical technology (for diagnosing, monitoring, testing, or

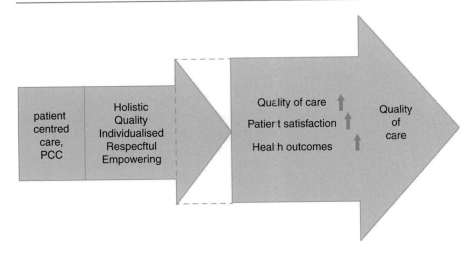

Fig. 25.2 Patient-centered care and quality of care. (After: Morgan and Yoder 2012)

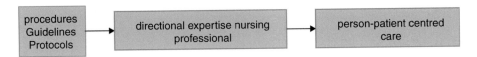

Fig. 25.3 Directing expertise of the nurse professional

administering patient treatments), information technology (such as records, using information and data to deliver care and document patient data), and knowledge technology (such as expert systems that can support decision-making about patient care). This can support nurses' clinical reasoning.

After all, a goal of quality of care is public information about health care. Based on it, people are offered insight into the quality of care and treatment provided in a particular health care facility. It contributes to enabling people to choose the health care facility where they would prefer to be treated.

Professionals should fill the professional space by providing their care from their vision of professional practice. This is not always easy, but it is a prerequisite for healthcare. We can distinguish two dimensions as extremes of each other:

- The first dimension is characterized by the nursing professional who works from her expertise to provide good quality care by performing care-related (partial) actions arising from guidelines and protocols.
- The second dimension is characterized by the nursing professional who takes charge of her own expertise and from this directing expertise provides care that is appropriate to the patient, person-centered care (Fig. 25.3).

Doing good in healthcare requires nursing professionals to think critically. However, the path to quality care is anything but one-dimensional. While the quality of care has certainly improved tremendously thanks to a variety of quality systems and by using evidence-based interventions, critical thinking by nursing professionals remains essential. To provide good care to the patient, it is important that, as a nurse, you have insight into what has proven to be effective care and treatment. It is important to be knowledgeable about the guidelines and protocols written for your patient group. But it takes a critical eye to assess what care is appropriate for THIS patient. It involves the critical eye of the nurse, combined with the needs of the patient, his unique situation psychologically, socially, and physically, with the insights from guidelines and research. By integrating these different dimensions into one's nursing practice, care can flourish.

In our health care system, there is a need to combine good care outcomes, with the need to keep the cost of that care as low as possible. The goal is to provide both effective and safe care, with the patient experience a key pillar of the quality of care. However, patients more often experience care as fragmented and discontinuous, and their patient needs are not always anticipated with care offerings (Naef et al. 2019).

Care should increasingly be patient-orchestrated care.

At the level of healthcare organization, validated and clinically relevant measurement tools are used. Patient Reported Outcome Measures (PROMs) are about outcomes of care that only patients can make reliable statements about. PROMs reported by patients include itching, side effects of medication, pain, shortness of breath, fatigue, and quality of life in general. We also distinguish Patient Reported Experience Measures (PREMs), which measure in a structured way how patients experience the quality of care (including relational aspects such as respectful engagement). PREMs are used to measure the effects and effectiveness of care and these results are used to improve care.

When quality awareness is established and there is a better understanding of what constitutes good care from relational caregiving and nursing, this is another way to look at quality of care.

The topic of quality of care comes up frequently while discussing quality systems. Quality management systems are used to improve the standard of care. It is common practice to use protocols, guidelines, and procedures in quality management systems. Quality is heavily influenced by the purposefulness and focus of the organization providing the care. Are patients aware of this, do they also have quality awareness just like professionals?

It is certainly true that today's patient wants to receive effective and efficient care. It is important for patients that this care is not only effective and efficient, but also patient specific. Patients want—and increasingly expect—that the care fits their specific (health) situation. This manifests itself on many levels. They want an appointment that fits into their agenda. They do not want general information, but specific health information about their specific situation. They want to be informed specifically what this means for them in their individual situation. They want cohesive, integrated care, with a certain user-friendliness and safety. Patients also expect healthcare providers to treat them with care as patients. Expertise and clarity are valued by patients, as is a certain degree of flexibility and cohesion between the care units provided. These are all aspects of care quality (Boot 2018).

Nursing professionals should use themselves as a tool to optimize the quality of care (Baart 2018). To this end, healthcare providers should:

- Learn to observe, assess, and improve the quality of care yourself;
- Enter into a relationship with the care recipients on site by allowing them to participate in the discussion;
- Have to frequently test (reflect) on the work floor and consult with colleagues in order to discover the good quality.

Peer review is a valuable tool for improving the quality of care. In peer reviews, the care is discussed on the basis of criteria for good care. By "examining" their own actions, useful information is obtained to optimize care in terms of goal-directedness and efficiency from the patient's perspective. How can we tailor the care to the individual patient, so that he or she feels seen and known and experiences the care provided as good? In the cyclical process of quality improvement, the quality is also determined by the patient. Quality promotion is then about taking the care experienced by patients into account in the quality cycle.

For good quality of care, it is important that care is offered in a cohesive range and that there is continuity in the care offer (Davis et al. 2005). Continuity and coordination of care are key elements of the quality of care. The nursing model of primary nursing does not seem to meet this requirement, and continuity and coordination should be improved by emphasizing relational, collaborative care (Naef et al. 2019). Nursing should therefore start more from establishing a relationship with the patient, to plan and coordinate care throughout the care process. Fragmentation can be avoided in this way, and more emphasis is placed on person-centered, high-quality nursing.

The quality of care can be improved through good coordination of (specialist) care. This is possible if there are systems in place that prevent errors in cases where multiple healthcare professionals are involved with the patient. For example, diagnostic tests that are done once and whose results are then used by multiple professionals. Systems focused on post-hospital follow-up and support, on tracking tests and test results, but also on communication between healthcare professionals who all contribute to the care of an individual patient, at different times and locations (Davis et al. 2005).

Continuity of care touches on a number of aspects of care (Maizes et al. 2009):

- Continuity of care implies that the healthcare provider is a familiar point of contact (a familiar face) for the patient or client, in the patient's contacts with the healthcare system. Ideally, each patient has his own healthcare provider as a contact person. This can be achieved in certain healthcare settings; in the case of a district nurse, for example, she may be the only professional who provides continuous care. More often, however, a team of professionals is focused on providing continuous care. A relationship with the patient is then established by examining and then integrating his personal needs and choices into the care plan. These are then implemented by the entire team.

- Continuity of care is also related to the availability of up-to-date and complete patient data. All professionals involved must have access to this.
- Continuity of care is also about ensuring a continuous care process from the start of the disease process to the end of the recovery process. The focus of healthcare is shifting from intramural healthcare from hospitals to extramural healthcare as close as possible to home (Yoder-Wisse 2019).
- Finally, continuity of care can be about entering into a contract with the patient stating which healthcare professional is responsible for the patient and his care, and who maintains contact with the patient's family.

Communicating for Continuity of Care (COC) is a term that emphasizes the importance of patient-centered quality care being about continuity of care and coordination of care, both within and across clinical settings (Haggerty et al. 2013; Arnold and Underman Boggs 2020). COC is about continuity and coordination in the relational field, about providing information specifically for people with chronic health problems. This goes a step further than the Chronic Care model, which talks about fostering productive relationships between informed patients plus family and prepared proactive practice teams.

Continuity of care delivered by a team of professionals supports the patient's recovery process. It offers professionals and patients the opportunity to build a relationship of trust, an alliance. By entering into the relationship or alliance, the patient's trust in the treatment may increase. This trusting relationship can encourage the patient to openly discuss their concerns. This relationship of trust also promotes adherence and self-management of the patient. It also has the positive effects that there is less acute care, less specialist care, fewer days of hospitalization and patient satisfaction is increasing in the direction of perfect care (Maizes et al. 2009).

One of the goals of quality of care is patient safety. Improving and monitoring patient safety is the responsibility of the entire team. In a systematic review, it appears that patients can participate in improving patient safety. This participation consists of informing professionals and pointing out negative effects or mistakes. This patient participation in patient safety has the advantage that the patient takes on an active role and is therefore more involved in his own care (Vaismoradi and Kangasniemi 2014).

Another goal of quality of care is patient-centered research. Patient-centered research is the routine collection of feedback from (a specific group of) patients to understand how care, treatment, and health care provision are experienced (Davis et al. 2005). This is to be able to assess what went right and wrong in the care from the patient's perspective. From here we can look at how the care can be improved and how the involvement of the patient can be improved. When patients feel involved in care and treatment, they are more likely to be adherent, they have a better understanding of their own health status, they experience a better quality of life and patient satisfaction is higher.

Finally, a goal of quality of care is public information about health care. On this basis, people are offered insight into the quality of the care and treatment provided in a particular healthcare facility or people can choose a particular healthcare facility.

25.5   Conclusion

- Quality of life is not only linked to physical health, but also to autonomy, emotional and relational aspects, and independent functioning. Patients' own assessment of their quality of life is essential for quality of care, which should be patient-centered and involve shared decision-making. The pillars of quality of care are patient satisfaction, performance improvement, regulatory constraints, clinical effectiveness, and patient safety. Providing patient-centered care improves patients' perceived quality of care, their satisfaction with care, and their functional capabilities, which, in turn, contributes to their well-being and quality of life. The challenge remains to offer patient-centered care in a cost-effective manner and to close the gap between the care patients receive and the care they should receive.
- Providing quality care is a complex process that involves not only the healthcare organization, care processes, and clinical information systems but also the individual needs and preferences of the patient. To improve quality of care, it is important to focus on patient-centered care and promote productive interactions between patients and healthcare providers. Active and empowered patients can help identify gaps in care, and healthcare professionals need to continuously assess and reflect on their own actions to ensure quality care. By monitoring and improving the quality of care, healthcare organizations can promote patient satisfaction and better outcomes. Overall, providing quality care requires a relational approach that considers the fragility of life and focuses on building strong relationships between patients and healthcare professionals.
- Providing quality of care to patients is essential, and nursing professionals play a significant role in achieving this goal. While guidelines and protocols can be useful, critical thinking and a patient-centered approach are necessary to provide appropriate care to each patient. Patients expect healthcare providers to offer care that is effective, efficient, and tailored to their specific needs. Quality management systems can help improve the standard of care, but patients' experiences and opinions should be considered in the quality cycle. Coordination and continuity of care are crucial elements of quality care, and nursing professionals should emphasize relational, collaborative care to achieve these goals.
- Ultimately, the goal of healthcare should be to provide patient-orchestrated care that is both effective and safe, with a positive patient experience as a key component of quality care.

Box 25.2 Mind-Map Improving Quality of Care
Create a mind-map on improving quality of care.

Point out how nursing professionals can improve the quality of care from her individual position. Name aspects at the micro-level, at the meso-level, and at the macro-level.

Box 25.3 Mind-Map Patient Journey and Quality of Care
Create a mind-map. The treatment of the patient is a process of health complaints, through procedures, referrals, and treatments to the end of treatment, with the aim of quality of life and health gain. The patient journey.

Point out the treatment process, and how you can optimize this process by giving patient preferences a clear role? How do you do it?

Box 25.4 Mind-Map Optimizing Quality of Care
Make a mind-map on optimizing quality of care.

Point out what is necessary to optimize the quality of care.

Use: the micro/patient level, at the meso/team level, and at the macro/organization level. Indicate whether the factors are positive or negative.

Nursing and the Patient Journey

26

26.1 Topic List: The Patient Journey and Quality of Care

1. Patient mapping or patient journey, definition and importance in highlighting patient experience, link with good care from patient's perspective.
2. Patient journey within quality of care, indicating the route of a patient through healthcare system.
3. Importance of understanding patient journey for person-centered care and shared decision-making.
4. Process mapping in optimizing care process, purpose of process mapping in improving quality of care and limitations in focusing solely on performance improvement.
5. Redesigning patient pathway based on patient journey, benefits of using patient journey for efficient and effective care, and benefits of patient empowerment through choices and patient-specific information.
6. Valuing patient satisfaction in care process, importance of patient satisfaction as an integral part of medical protocols and guidelines.
7. Role of nurses in improving care through patient journey; impact of starting care from patient journey on efficiency and outcomes, and detection of errors and insight into overproduction and waiting times.
8. Continuum of care from a patient perspective, benefits of a care continuum, and consequences of gaps in healthcare provision and unmet patient needs.
9. Importance of patient journey in quality of care: the need for patient-centric approach in medical protocols, guidelines, and ethical standards.

B. Sassen, *Improving Person-Centered Innovation of Nursing Care*,
https://doi.org/10.1007/978-3-031-35048-1_26

26.2   Introduction

The healthcare system can be a complex and overwhelming experience for patients, especially when they are faced with illness or injury. To ensure that patients receive the best care possible, it is important to take their perspective into account when designing medical protocols and guidelines. This is where the concept of patient journey comes into play. Patient journey refers to the process a patient goes through within a health care facility or system as a whole.

By understanding the patient's journey, healthcare providers can identify areas that need improvement, such as inefficiencies or gaps in care, and make necessary changes to optimize the quality of care. The focus on patient satisfaction and empowerment can lead to better outcomes and higher patient satisfaction. Ultimately, the goal is to provide a continuum of care that is continuous and consistent with the needs, preferences, and expectations of the patient.

26.3   Topic

This chapter discusses the concept of patient journey, which is a tool used to understand and improve the patient experience within the healthcare system. It explains how patient journey differs from medical protocols or guidelines, which tend to prioritize treatment over the patient experience. The chapter also highlights the importance of patient satisfaction as a measure of quality of care, and how process mapping can be used to optimize the care process. It further emphasizes the benefits of viewing care from the patient's perspective, including greater efficiency and effectiveness, and the importance of continuity of care to ensure positive patient outcomes.

26.4   Patient Mapping or Patient Journey

A medical protocol or guideline consists of a set of treatment guidelines that describe what the treatment should look like; in this, the patient experience is usually secondary. Patient mapping or patient journey is a tool to better highlight this patient experience (McCarthy et al. 2016). The patient journey makes specific what contributes to good care and what does not—from the perspective of the patient or client.

Within quality of care, the concept of patient journey is also used to indicate the route that a patient takes through the healthcare system: from diagnosis, with successive interactions and contacts between the patient and the healthcare system (Elliss-Brookes et al. 2012). When we look at care from the patient's perspective and look at the process a patient has gone through within a health care facility or within the health care system, we speak of patient journey. For example, a patient journey is the process from admission for surgery or major depressive disorder to discharge.

The patient journey clarifies the complex phases that a patient goes through when he uses healthcare. Understanding this can make visible how person-centered care and shared decision-making can be better facilitated, how patient satisfaction can be improved, how patient participation can be improved and result in care and treatment and patient outcomes that meet the needs and wishes of patients. reflect (Gregory 2012).

Process mapping provides insight into whether the care process can be optimized. The purpose of process mapping is to get a picture of the process, and to see what attention—read improvement—needs to be done to improve the quality of care. The aim is to identify problems and based on this, to make suggestions for optimizing the quality of care (Trebble et al. 2010). However, the focus of process mapping is often mainly on performance improvement and regulatory constraints, and much less on patient satisfaction as a point of reference for improving the quality of care (Bate and Robert 2006; McCarthy et al. 2016).

By viewing a care process from the patient or client perspective, effectiveness and efficiency can be maximized by eliminating ineffective or unnecessary care. Viewing a patient journey can result in a redesign of the patient pathway: the entire care process can be adjusted accordingly. The revised care process is more efficient and effective, leading to greater patient satisfaction and quality of care (Trebble et al. 2010). By using a patient journey, choices can be offered in combination with patient-specific information—two important expressions of patient empowerment (McCarthy et al. 2016).

The focus here should also be on activities that are valued by patients, as they lead to higher patient satisfaction (Trebble et al. 2010).

If nurses start their care from the patient journey, this improves the efficiency and outcomes of care. For professionals, this leads to the detection of errors, for example, prescription errors regarding medication. But also, to insight into overproduction (unnecessary tests and treatments) and the length of waiting times (Trebble et al. 2010). Moreover, it would contribute to better care if patient satisfaction became an integral part of medical protocols, guidelines, and ethical standards (McCarthy et al. 2016).

From a patient perspective, a continuum of care would be preferable. A care continuum would consist of care that is continuous regarding the care providers involved: the same care provider(s) within the same healthcare organization maintain contact with "their" patient. If gaps arise in healthcare, this usually has an adverse effect on the results and outcomes of healthcare. Gaps can arise if the provision of care by one healthcare professional stops, while this is not picked up by another healthcare professional, while this is desirable in the context of effective care. Gaps can also arise if the healthcare provider does not sufficiently meet the needs, preferences, and expectations of the patient.

26.5   Conclusion

- The patient journey is a valuable tool for improving the quality of care by highlighting the patient's perspective and experience within the healthcare system.
- By mapping out the patient's journey, healthcare professionals can identify areas for improvement and optimize the care process to be more efficient and effective. It is crucial to focus on activities that are valued by patients, leading to higher patient satisfaction and better outcomes.
- Incorporating patient satisfaction as an integral part of medical protocols, guidelines, and ethical standards would contribute to better care.
- Additionally, a continuum of care with continuous contact with the same healthcare provider(s) would be preferable from a patient's perspective to avoid gaps in healthcare and ensure effective care.
- Ultimately, putting the patient at the center of the care process can lead to better care and outcomes that meet the needs and wishes of patients.

Box 26.1 Mind-Map The patient journey and patients' perspective What Contributes to Good Care

Create a mind-map on patient journey. The concept of patient journey is used to indicate the route a patient takes through the healthcare system

Use a specific route from a patient group with a specific health problem or disease and describe the route in steps.

And then highlight in this route the patient experience with care, and it makes clear from the patient's or client's perspective what contributes to good care and what does not.

What can (relatively easily) be changed in the patient journey to improve the quality of care?

Name 2 plus points for the patient/client group; name 2 plus points for healthcare professionals.

Box 26.2 Mind-Map Patient Journey, Process Mapping, and Care Continuum

Create a mind-map that visualizes the relationship between patient journey, quality of care, process mapping, and care continuum. Use this mind-map as a tool to analyze and identify areas for improvement in a healthcare facility of your choice.

Choose a healthcare facility (hospital, clinic, etc.) of your choice.

Use the information provided to create a mind-map that connects patient journey, quality of care, process mapping, and care continuum.

Use the mind-map to identify areas for improvement in the chosen healthcare facility.

Nursing and Triple Aim and Quadruple Aim

27.1 Topic List: Triple Aim and Quadruple Aim for Optimizing the Functioning of the Health Care System

1. Triple Aim and Quadruple Aim can be used to Improve patient experience: Enhancing patient satisfaction, engagement, and involvement in care through personalized and patient-centered approaches. Prioritizing patient preferences and values in decision-making processes.
2. For improving population health: Implementing strategies to address the health needs of diverse populations, promoting preventive care, health promotion, and disease management at the community and population levels.
3. For reducing costs: Implementing cost-effective measures, optimizing resource utilization, and promoting value-based care to reduce healthcare costs while maintaining quality outcomes.
4. For improving the work life of healthcare professionals: Addressing healthcare professional burnout, improving job satisfaction, and promoting work–life balance through supportive work environments, effective leadership, recognition, and staffing.
5. Partnering with patients as consumers: Encouraging engaged, equal partnerships between healthcare professionals and patients, based on trust, communication, and shared decision-making. Promoting patient empowerment, responsibility, and involvement in their own care.
6. Conditions for a healthy working environment: Fostering supported cooperation, effective decision-making, expert communication, leadership, professional recognition, and appropriate staffing to create a healthy work environment for healthcare professionals to thrive and deliver clinically excellent care.
7. Prioritization of healthcare professionals' health: Encouraging healthcare professionals to prioritize their own health and well-being through self-management, self-evaluation, and setting personal goals to manage work-related stress and enhance their involvement in patient care.

8. Care team well-being in the Quadruple Aim: Recognizing the well-being of the entire care team, including interdisciplinary collaboration, effective communication, and leadership, as essential for delivering optimal patient care and improving overall healthcare outcomes.

27.2   Outline

This chapter discusses the evolution of the Triple Aim in healthcare, which originally aimed to improve patient experience, population health, and reduce costs, but has now been extended to include a fourth goal of improving the work life of healthcare professionals, known as the Quadruple Aim. Burnout and dissatisfaction among healthcare professionals can lead to reduced patient satisfaction, so the Quadruple Aim emphasizes the need to prioritize the health and well-being of healthcare professionals. To achieve this, healthcare professionals must carry out targeted self-management and prioritize their own health.

Additionally, a healthy working environment with supported cooperation, effective decision-making, expert communication, leadership, professional recognition, and good staffing is essential. Partnering with patients as consumers is also important for optimizing the quality of the healthcare system, and this requires an engaged, equal relationship based on trust and careful listening by healthcare professionals to patients. The chapter emphasizes the importance of healthcare professionals' well-being in achieving clinically excellent care and optimal patient outcomes.

27.3   Introduction

The Triple Aim is a well-known framework in healthcare that aims to optimize the functioning of the healthcare system by improving patient experience, population health, and reducing costs. However, healthcare professionals are also an essential part of this system, and their well-being is crucial for the provision of quality care. Therefore, the Quadruple Aim was introduced, which adds a fourth goal: improving the work life of healthcare professionals. This paper explores the importance of the well-being of healthcare professionals in achieving the Quadruple Aim and the role of partnering with patients as consumers in optimizing the functioning of the healthcare system.

27.4   Optimizing the Functioning of Healthcare

Triple aim purposes to optimize the functioning of the health care system. It is about improving patient experience, improving population health, and reducing costs. The quadruple aim adds a fourth goal: improving the work life of healthcare professionals (Bodenheimer and Sinsky 2014).

Care professionals do not always experience the current health care system as pleasant. Dissatisfaction and burnout occur above average, also among nursing professionals. This requires attention, because burnout of professionals appears to lead to reduced patient and client satisfaction with the care provided. This has resulted in more and more attention being paid to the position of healthcare professionals, and the triple aim has been extended to the quadruple aim.

The quadruple aim emphasizes that care for patients demands care for professionals:

Care of the patient requires care of the provider (Bodenheimer and Sinsky 2014).

The aim is to improve the health of professionals, thus increasing their involvement in the provision of care and limiting turnover (Baum 2021). According to Baum (2021), this means that healthcare professionals should also take good care of their own health and carry out targeted self-management, giving priority to their own health. For this self-management and prioritization of one's own health, healthcare professionals should know their own response to stressful events and respond to this with self-evaluation. They should know their own goals, ranked by priority, and focus on them as work pressure increases.

If the goal is to generate optimal patient outcomes in healthcare, clinically excellent care is essential. And clinically excellent care can only be provided if healthcare professionals are able to perform under optimal conditions. A healthy working environment is an essential prerequisite for this. After all, the well-being of healthcare professionals also depends on a healthy work environment.

In order to be able to speak of a healthy working environment, the following conditions must be met (Fig. 27.1):

- Supported cooperation (true collaboration);
- Effective decision-making;
- Expert communication (skilled communication);
- Leadership;
- Professional recognition (meaningful recognition);
- Good staffing (appropriate staffing).

In the quadruple aim it is about (Fig. 27.2):

1. The patient experience;
2. Health of groups in society (population health);
3. Reducing costs;
4. The well-being of the professional team (care team well-being).

When it comes to improving healthcare, partnering with the patient as a consumer is also an option. Partnering with consumers is an important element in optimizing the functioning, and therefore the quality, of the health care system. A patient who

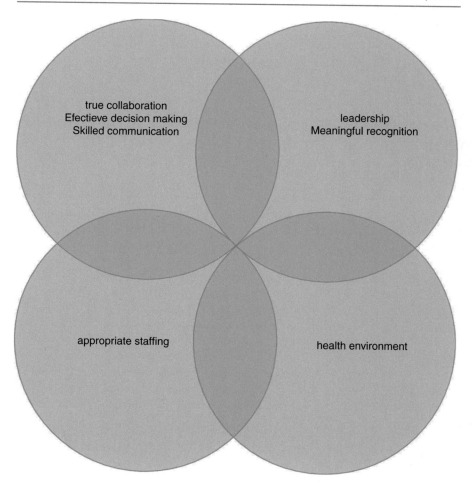

Fig. 27.1 Excellent care. (According to: Describing Nurse Leaders' and Direct Care Nurses 2016)

gives a low assessment of the extent to which he is approached as a partner in care will also rate the quality of care as low (Gill and Gill 2015).

For partnerships, an engaged, equal relationship with the patient or client is important, based on trust and careful listening by the professional to the patient or client. The professional can relinquish and transfer responsibility if the patient (or patient group) accepts greater responsibility. As a result, patients gain more control and responsibility for individual choices. But this partnership also extends further to advisory committees, health care facilities, and possibly the health care sector. The point is that "consumers"—patients and clients in the case of healthcare—use this freedom to respond to their needs and values, but also see this as a shared responsibility (Gill and Gill 2015).

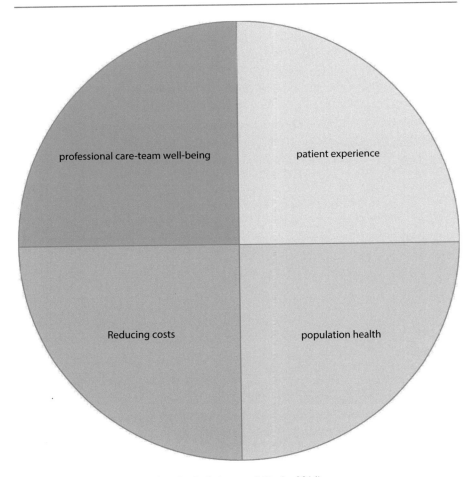

Fig. 27.2 Quadruple aim. (After: Bodenheimer and Sinsky 2014)

27.5   Conclusion

- The patient journey is a valuable tool for improving the quality of care by highlighting the patient's perspective and experience within the healthcare system.
- By mapping out the patient's journey, healthcare professionals can identify areas for improvement and optimize the care process to be more efficient and effective. It is crucial to focus on activities that are valued by patients, leading to higher patient satisfaction and better outcomes.
- Incorporating patient satisfaction as an integral part of medical protocols, guidelines, and ethical standards would contribute to better care.

- Additionally, a continuum of care with continuous contact with the same healthcare provider(s) would be preferable from a patient's perspective to avoid gaps in healthcare and ensure effective care.
- Ultimately, putting the patient at the center of the care process can lead to better care and outcomes that meet the needs and wishes of patients.

Box 27.1 Mind-Map The *Quadruple Aim*
In the quadruple aim it is emphasized that care for patients requires care for professionals (care of the patient requires care of the provider).
Point out how this can be done better (in the setting where you work)?

Box 27.2 Mind-Map Quadruple Aim Healthcare Professionals' Well-Being
Create a mind-map exploring the quadruple aim in healthcare and how it relates to healthcare professionals' well-being and patient care.
Use these elements:

- The quadruple aim: Improving patient experience, improving population health, reducing costs, and improving the work life of healthcare professionals.
- The importance of healthcare professionals' well-being in providing quality patient care.
- Conditions necessary for a healthy working environment, including supported cooperation, effective decision-making, expert communication, leadership, professional recognition, and good staffing.
- The importance of partnering with patients as consumers to optimize the functioning of the healthcare system.
- Elements of a successful patient partnership, including an engaged, equal relationship based on trust and careful listening by the professional, and the transfer of responsibility to patients who accept greater responsibility.

Use colors, symbols, and images to organize and connect the different elements. Consider adding examples or case studies to illustrate your points.

Nursing and Patient-Centered Leadership

28

28.1 Topic List: Nurses as Leaders in Healthcare

1. Importance of nurses in the healthcare system, pivotal role in the health care system, and should take the lead to drive change for their patients and patient care.
2. Leadership in healthcare, a basic attitude of nurses, need for direct involvement in clinical care while constantly influencing others to improve care, and need for empowerment and creating a consistent focus on the needs of patients.
3. Leadership skills can be acquired by any nursing professional, contrary to the idea that it is a personality trait. Communication, collaboration, team building, and other interpersonal skills as foundation of nursing leadership and management.
4. Positive relationship between relational leadership and patient satisfaction, and a strong relationship between leadership and patient safety processes.
5. Goals of nursing leadership are challenging others to provide patient-centered care, building partnerships with patients and families, and raising and maintaining efficient and effective care to increase patient satisfaction and quality of care.
6. Different leadership styles in healthcare.
7. Importance of professionalism in nursing leadership, moving from obedient professionals to sensible professionals, and evidence-based knowledge, skillful action, and right skills for carrying out the nursing profession.
8. Benefits of transformational leadership: Connecting with ideals of patient-centered care; enhancing the patient experience; and building bridges to effective and/or innovative care outcomes.
9. Patient-centered leadership, acquisition of leadership qualities by every nurse needs; empowering and motivating others to provide patient-centered care; being visionary and creating professional care from a vision; and importance of communication, cooperation, coaching, and monitoring in leadership skills.

B. Sassen, *Improving Person-Centered Innovation of Nursing Care*, https://doi.org/10.1007/978-3-031-35048-1_28

28.2   Topics

This chapter discusses the importance of nursing leadership in the healthcare system. It emphasizes the need for nurses to take the lead in driving change for their patients and patient care. The chapter also mentions the acquisition of leadership skills, which can be acquired by any nurse, and the competences that make up nursing leadership and management, such as communication, collaboration, and team building.

The text also highlights the positive relationship between relational leadership and patient satisfaction, leading to fewer medication errors, fewer hospital infections, and lower mortality. It describes the different leadership styles, including relational, task-oriented, supportive, situational, transactional, and transformational leadership, and how they can be combined for effective care. The text also emphasizes the need for nurses to possess evidence-based knowledge and insights about desired care, as well as the right skills to carry out their profession. Finally, the text describes the move from obedient professionals to sensible professionals and the importance of professionalism in nursing.

28.3   Introduction

Nursing professionals are essential members of the healthcare team who play a critical role in providing patient-centered care. With their direct involvement in clinical care and constant influence on others, nurses have the opportunity to drive positive change for their patients and for healthcare as a whole. Leadership is a fundamental aspect of nursing, and every nurse has the ability to acquire leadership skills. Effective nursing leadership involves a combination of interpersonal and communication skills that form the foundation of nursing management. In this essay, we will explore the importance of patient-centered leadership in nursing and how it can improve patient outcomes.

Providing relational care and acquiring quality awareness demands professionalism from nurses, and this requires patient-oriented leadership. According to Baart (2018), this requires a different kind of professionalism, where nurses should seek and discover the good in relational care repeatedly. In addition to evidence-based knowledge, nurses must possess the right skills to carry out their profession.

This text highlights the importance of nursing leadership in providing optimal patient care. The author argues that nurses should adopt a patient-centered approach and take responsibility for the entire care patient journey of their patients. Furthermore, the chapter emphasizes the need for a multidisciplinary approach and the importance of tailoring interventions to individual patient needs. The author also highlights the need for nurses to be flexible in their leadership styles and to show leadership in situations where protocols and guidelines obstruct the view of what is right or wise to do. Overall, the text emphasizes the critical role of nursing leadership in improving the quality of care and the quality of life of patient and client groups.

28.4 Leadership for Change

Nurses should play a pivotal role in the health care system. They need to seize opportunities and take the lead to drive change for their patients and patient care. It is the task of nurses to ensure that the focus in care and treatment is on patient-centered, relational care and to ensure that care is accessible, cost-effective, and high-quality, result-oriented care (Yoder 2019).

Leadership in healthcare can be described as the basic attitude of nurses (Giltinane 2013):

> Direct involvement in clinical care while constantly influencing others to improve the care they are providing

And:

> [...] to empower and create a consistent focus on the needs of patients.

Patient-centered leadership is the acquisition of leadership qualities, and every nurse can acquire these leadership skills. Leadership can be acquired by any nursing professional, contrary to the idea that it is a personality trait (Cummings et al. 2008).

Leadership consists of several competences that you can acquire (Fischer 2016). Communication, collaboration, team building, and other interpersonal skills form the foundation of nursing leadership and management (Fig. 28.1; Yoder 2019).

In an update of a systematic review, it appears that there is a positive relationship between relational leadership and patient satisfaction. This review showed that relational leadership led to more patient satisfaction with care, but also led to fewer medication errors, fewer hospital infections, and lower mortality (Wong et al. 2013). In fact, there is a strong relationship between leadership and patient safety processes (Thompson 2012).

The goal of nursing leadership is to challenge others to provide patient-centered care, building partnerships with the patient and family. The goal of nursing leadership is also to raise and maintain efficient and effective care to increase patient satisfaction and the quality of care (Giltinane 2013).

Relational leadership strengthens organizational strategies and improves care outcomes (Wong et al. 2013).

Leadership skills include (Kouzes and Posner 2008):

- Setting a good example;
- Empowering and motivating others to provide patient-centered care;
- Be visionary and create professional care from your vision;
- Communicate, cooperate, coach, and monitor.

Providing relational care and acquiring quality awareness demands professionalism from nurses and this requires patient-oriented leadership.

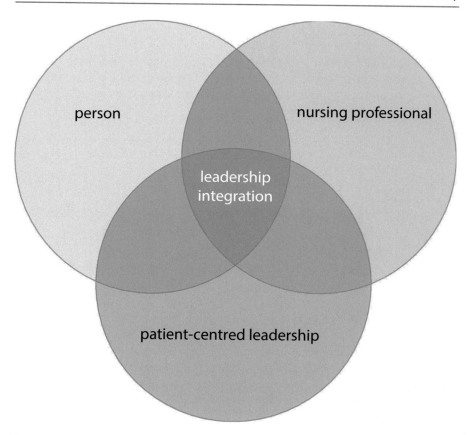

Fig. 28.1 Integrating roles to achieve nursing leadership. (After: Yoder 2019)

According to Baart (2018), it requires a different kind of professionalism. This means that the good must always be scoped by the nurse. The good in relational care must be sought and discovered over and over again.

Sensible professionals should take as a starting point: "this seems like a good thing to do" (Baart 2018). Nurses should have evidence-based knowledge and insights about what is desired in the care and which care has been proven to be effective. In addition to this knowledge, nurses must be able to act skillfully and possess the right skills that professionals need to carry out their profession.

According to Baart (2018), healthcare professionals must move from obedient professionals to sensible professionals. The current complaisance eventually extinguishes your moral sense, making it increasingly difficult to see when the care is no longer good. You no longer see that it is not the right treatment for the patient, that the good care is not provided, that the patient's needs are not met, or that the patient is lonely.

We can distinguish different leadership styles (Fig. 28.2). Leadership styles can differ from each other because they have a different focus (Cummings et al. 2008).

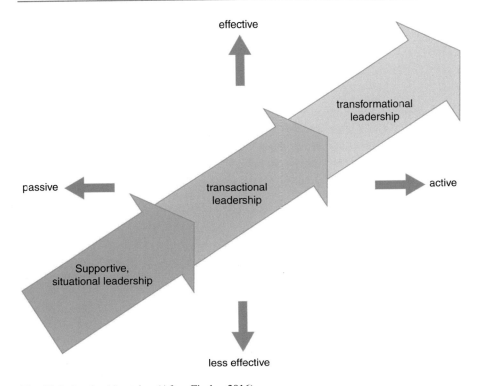

Fig. 28.2 Leadership styles. (After: Fischer 2016)

1. As a healthcare professional, you can have a relational orientation and focus on people and the relationships between people. As a professional, you can also have a task orientation and focus on organizational structures and tasks. Both leadership styles are important for the smooth running of care processes (Wong et al. 2013).

    Relational leadership requires emotional competences from nurses, creating a positive atmosphere in the care setting. Nurses can offer support and encouragement, provide positive and constructive feedback. The communication is open and transparent, with a high level of individual involvement of the healthcare professional. An important element of relational leadership is that it entails entering a dialogue with others, both with patients and with colleagues.

    Relational leadership should be combined with task-oriented leadership, with an emphasis on the execution and monitoring of the tasks. The combination of both leadership styles is referred to as transactional leadership.

2. Supportive leadership is experienced as pleasant because it is based on open communication and offering emotional support. Situational leadership is attractive because different situations call for a different way of taking charge. This is in contrast to directive leadership, in which tasks are explained and assigned, which is more often experienced as unpleasant and as an infringement of professional autonomy (Giltinane 2013).

3. Transactional leadership places the emphasis on the interaction between team members. For patients, this increases patient satisfaction, as well as patient safety. This by knowing the patient needs and implementing effective interventions in order to provide effective safe care (Tregunno et al. 2009).

4. Transformationeel leiderschap bestaat uit een manier van communiceren die een verbinding legt met idealen over hoe de zorg eruit zou moeten zien en hoe er patiëntgecentreerde zorg kan worden verleend. Dit biedt professionals een emotionele betrokkenheid, wat hen extra motiveert in hun werk. Transformational leadership emphasizes participation. Transformational leadership is intellectually challenging, inspiring, and motivating. Bridges are built to effective and/or innovative care outcomes (Bass et al. 2003). Transformational leadership by nurses can enhance the patient experience (Kutney-Lee et al. 2016). For the profession itself, transformational leadership leads to high-performing teams, and this improves patient care, including patient safety (Fischer 2016). This form of leadership is experienced as reliable and authentic (Fischer 2016). Transformational leadership consists of a way of communicating that connects to ideals about what care should look like and how patient-centered care can be delivered. This offers healthcare professionals an emotional involvement, which motivates them even more in their work.

According to Giltinane (2013), leadership is mainly about being flexible in leadership styles, the leadership style used then depends on the context. Good leadership is about integrating diverse leadership styles.

Sensible professionals should break the tendency that patient-specific factors underlie non-compliance with the treatment plan. The focus of professionals is now often that patients do not follow the recommendations, but…:

Patients need to be supported, not blamed (WHO 2003).

Nurses should show leadership in a broadly supported perspective of de-blaming across the profession. No evidence has been found in the literature that there is an association between patient-specific factors and adherence to the recommendations associated with care and treatment. However, the health care system as a whole, with the way in which health care professionals operate in it, is related to following the recommendations that accompany care and treatment (WHO 2003).

Transformational leadership skills are appropriate for nurses. Thompson lists the following three transformational leadership skills (Thompson 2012):

1. Professionals must work together in an empowering way, enabling colleagues to learn and adopt a transformational leadership style.
2. Turning evidence into practice, and subsequently turning practice into evidence.
3. Critically reflective working and communicating, problem-solving thinking and acting, and decision-making.

The degree to which patients can feel that they are part of the care and treatment plan is determined by socio-economic factors, the health team and health care system, and the characteristics of the patient's or client's health problem. It takes leadership from nurses to make the patient part of the health team, considering the characteristics of the health problem and the biopsychosocial health of the patient.

Nurses should show leadership in distinguishing situations where quality of care needs to be tailored, and situations where this is debatable or not visible. It takes nursing leadership to detect the gaps in care and identify the "bugs" for patients in the care pathway, in the care system, or in the delivery of care. These gaps and pitfalls can cause real problems for patients and can even be seen as pain points in the health care system.

Care is to detect these pain points and to handle them adequately, so that they become easy to manage for the patient. By recognizing and subsequently analyzing the causes of these bugs in the healthcare system, nurses can work toward reducing or eliminating them and thereby improving the quality of care. Nursing leadership is required for this, both in detecting and analyzing the pain points, working toward solutions in a multidisciplinary manner, and working toward the implementation of solutions in patient care. Such a form of nursing leadership can lead to quality improvements in care delivery, in the quality of care and in the organization of healthcare as a whole and in the quality of life of patient and client groups.

A multidisciplinary approach can boost the handling of the pain points and lead to the elimination of the bugs in care and treatment. Nursing leadership is an indispensable pillar for properly embedding relational care in nursing care. And by simultaneously developing this in a multidisciplinary manner, the quality of care can improve further. This requires coordinated action by healthcare professionals, but also by policy makers in and outside the healthcare sector.

It requires a learning organization to achieve optimal quality assurance. There is no single or simple intervention or strategy that is appropriate for all patients, in all circumstances, and for all settings. Interventions always require focusing on the specific patient group and on the specific patient needs. Interventions should be tailored to individual patients. Interventions should be specifically tailored to the disease-specific needs of the patient. It requires patient-oriented leadership from nurses to organize care in such a way that these disease-specific needs are always the starting point of care provision. And, that factors that influence these patient needs, insofar as they arise or persist, are included in this. We call this professional development (Fig. 28.3).

Nurses should also show leadership in taking responsibility, where responsibility should be understood as a professional responsibility. No longer "looking away" when person-centered, integrated care is compromised, but take responsibility for this. If the goal is to provide relational care, aimed at optimizing the patient's quality of life, it is an important element of patient-centered leadership to also take explicit responsibility for this. Nursing leadership is taking responsibility for (keeping an eye on) the whole patient, for the patient's entire care path, from the beginning to the aftercare of the treatment. Think of a child in the fourth grade of secondary education with eating disorders and who is "looking" for suitable care and treatment together with her parent. The parent is strongly involved with her child, she also

Fig. 28.3 Professional
development

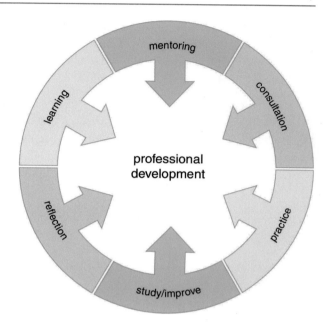

experiences stress as a result and therefore suffers from sleep disorders. In this case, taking responsibility means not looking away from the parent's health problems, but also paying specific attention to them, in addition to caring for the child.

Nurses should show leadership in situations where protocols and guidelines obstruct the view of what is right to do or obstruct the view of what is wise to do (Baart 2018). For their professional development, it is important that nursing professionals provide targeted input so that they can continue to act up-to-date and professionally. And the fact that they continue to play an active role in this, we call this professional action (Fig. 28.4).

Nurses should be able to account for and weigh up their actions. They need to reflect on their way of providing care. Always ask yourself the question: What is the best thing to do, in this situation, with this patient (group) and in this context? It is important to reflect on the good, but this always depends on the context in which the care is provided. It requires enthusiasm and responsibility on the part of the professional to ensure that care in the context matches the needs of the patient (Baart 2018).

Baart (2018) mentions that it requires a leap: nurses should take a leap and think "I'm going to do it." To the best of my knowledge, this is a good thing to do and not to do!

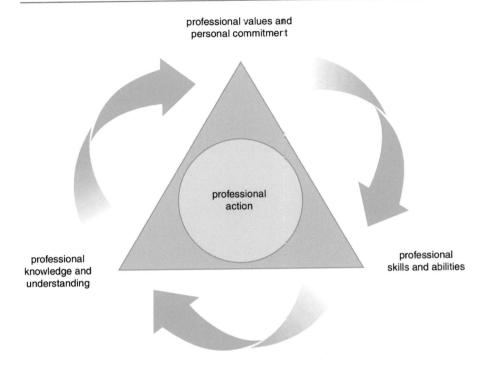

Fig. 28.4 Professional action

28.5 Conclusion

- Patient-centered leadership is crucial for improving patient outcomes and providing high-quality care. Nurses have the ability to acquire leadership skills and influence positive change for their patients and the healthcare system as a whole.
- Effective nursing leadership involves setting a good example, empowering and motivating others, being visionary, and communicating, cooperating, coaching, and monitoring. By strengthening organizational strategies and building partnerships with patients and their families, nurses can achieve patient-centered care and improve patient satisfaction.
- It is imperative that nursing leadership be integrated into clinical practice to improve patient safety and care outcomes.
- Different leadership styles can be used in healthcare settings, and the combination of relational and task-oriented leadership, known as transactional leadership, is crucial for the smooth running of care processes. Transformational leadership, which emphasizes participation, idealizes patient-centered care, and motivates healthcare professionals, can lead to high-performing teams, improving patient

care, including patient safety. Sensible professionalism is required from healthcare professionals, which should always aim for the good in relational care and possess the necessary skills and knowledge to carry out their profession effectively.

- It is essential for nurses to exhibit transformational leadership skills, show responsibility, and take charge of patient care for quality improvements.
- Nurses need to be able to account for their actions and reflect on the best course of action for patients. Multidisciplinary approaches and patient-oriented leadership are indispensable in providing optimal quality assurance.
- By recognizing and addressing the gaps and pitfalls in healthcare, nursing leadership can lead to quality improvements in care delivery and the quality of life of patients and client groups.
- Therefore, nurses should continue to develop their skills and play an active role in professional development and action, contributing to up-to-date and professional healthcare.

Box 28.1 Mind-Map Leadership Styles
Create a mind-map. Establish relationships between patient-centered leadership and leadership styles. You indicate for each factor which leadership style it belongs to. And you indicate where you feel most comfortable.

Box 28.2 Mind-Map Nursing Leadership and Patient-Centered Care
Create a mind-map on the topic "Nursing Leadership and Patient-Centered Care." Use the information provided in the text, including the definition of nursing leadership, the competencies required for nursing leadership, the different leadership styles, and the importance of patient-centered care.
  Your mind-map should include the following:

1. Definition of nursing leadership
2. Competencies required for nursing leadership
3. Importance of patient-centered care
4. Different leadership styles
5. Relational leadership
6. Task-oriented leadership
7. Transactional leadership
8. Transformational leadership
9. Positive outcomes of nursing leadership

10. Empowerment of nurses to drive change in patient care
11. Professionalism and sensibility in nursing care
12. The role of communication in nursing leadership

You can use colors, images, and keywords to make your mind-map more engaging and informative. Make sure to include all the main ideas and details in a clear and organized way.

Nursing and Value-Based Healthcare 29

29.1 Topic List: Healthcare and the Use of Big Data

1. Value-Based Healthcare and the Use of Big Data.
2. Principles of Value-Based Healthcare: Patient as a Consumer, Focus on Recovery, Multidisciplinary Approach.
3. Measuring Patient Outcomes in Value-Based Healthcare.
4. Role of Data Collection in Understanding Care Outcomes.
5. Cost-Containment in Healthcare through Value-Based Approach.
6. Improving Care Efficiency through Value-Based Healthcare.
7. Nursing Leadership in Patient-Oriented Care.
8. Feedback and Improvement of Nursing Care in Value-Based Healthcare.
9. Impact of Value-Based Healthcare on Chronic Health Conditions.
10. Ensuring High-Quality Nursing Care in Value-Based Healthcare.

29.2 Outline

This chapter describes the concept of value-based healthcare, which is an approach that focuses on improving patient care and healthcare based on big data. This approach involves measuring the impact of care for a specific patient and collecting data to gain insight into the care outcomes and patient outcomes of care. The emphasis is on outcomes, and the patient's experienced quality of life is a primary consideration. Value-based healthcare aims to limit healthcare costs by avoiding unnecessary care and treatment, shortening treatments and care, and making care and treatment less invasive for the patient. Nursing patient-oriented leadership is crucial in implementing changes to care processes and providing effective and high-quality nursing care.

B. Sassen, *Improving Person-Centered Innovation of Nursing Care*,
https://doi.org/10.1007/978-3-031-35048-1_29

29.3   Introduction

The current healthcare system is driven by diagnosis classifications and treatment combinations, with emphasis placed on healthcare performance within a healthcare performance model. However, a value-based orientation in healthcare is a recent development that focuses on improving patient care and healthcare as a whole based on big data.

It aims to measure the impact of care for a specific patient and improve care outcomes by making changes to the input. This approach is patient-centered and considers the patient's perspective in every decision made about care and treatment.

29.4   Valuae-Based Patient-Centered Care

In our current healthcare system, diagnosis classifications hold significant sway. Upon receiving a diagnosis, a corresponding treatment plan is developed while taking care performance into account. This approach emphasizes healthcare performance within a performance model, with the starting point for care and treatment being a cluster of comparable disorders, based on their nature and severity rather than the specific diagnosis of the patient or client. As a result, funding is determined by the care demand, which prioritizes the needs of the patient or client (Cleary et al. 2012a, b).

To fully embrace a value-based orientation in healthcare, it is imperative to prioritize the patient's perspective in all decisions related to their care and treatment. This requires moving beyond mere assumptions and involving the patient in a collaborative decision-making process that considers the medical-technical options available, as well as the patient's unique interests and experiences. In situations where there is a clash of values, it is vital to show mutual respect and engage in open discussion of different viewpoints to find the optimal solution for the patient (Cleary et al. 2012a, b).

For nurses, value-based healthcare—i.e. care driven by values—is a fairly recent development.

Value-based healthcare is about how you can improve patient care and healthcare as a whole on the basis of big data (Porter et al. 2013; Ying et al. 2016). Based on data collected on a large scale, an attempt is made to further optimize the quality of care after analyzing this data. By collecting data from patients and analyzing this data, we gain more insight into the care outcomes, the patient outcomes of care. We have a better idea of which input leads to which output for the patient. This may not sound like a good fit for healthcare, but within the professional space in the healthcare process, patient-oriented care remains important and indispensable for good quality healthcare.

Important principles associated with a value-based orientation on care are that the patient as a consumer is central to the organizational goals, that the focus is on recovery rather than on treatment per se, and finally, a principle that good quality care requires a multidisciplinary approach to care and treatment.

Value-based healthcare is about outcomes, patient outcomes of care and treatment. The starting point here should be that the patient's experienced quality of life will increase as a result. Care and treatment should be directed toward achieving a favorable health outcome. The health outcome is as optimal as possible, considering the health situation of the patient and his quality of life. When you are ill, you expect everything to be about getting better (Cleary et al. 2012a, b).

With value-based healthcare you try to measure the impact of care for a specific patient. You then collect data from this specific patient, for example, someone with diabetes or someone with depression. For example, for an elementary school-aged child with diabetes who receives an insulin pump, you measure his blood glucose levels monthly for a year, you measure his well-being and perceived quality of life four times during a year, you measure his self-management skills four times during the year, and you read the data from the App used by the child. Or, for example, in the case of a person in his 20s with depressive symptoms who has to take medication, the degree of well-being and perceived quality of life are measured, you measure his blood levels with regard to the medication and you read the data from the App about the remind function. for taking medication and being physically active. By collecting this data, we gain more insight into the process between the input (start with the treatment or care) and the output (the result of the care and treatment provided). The data is collected from a specific group of patients or clients; data is viewed at the group level. With a better understanding of this process, care outcomes may be improved by making changes to the input.

In healthcare, much is aimed at reducing costs and at least keeping the quality of care the same. Value-based healthcare is also a way to limit healthcare costs. We all know that if our efforts are not focused on limiting health care expenditures, expenditures will become uncontrollable. In that regard, value-based healthcare can aim to improve treatment and care by:

– To avoid care and treatment,
– To avoid unnecessary actions and procedures,
– To shorten treatments and care, and
– To make care and treatment less invasive for the patient.

For example, if patients receive specific care so that they require less aftercare and can be discharged sooner. Or, if patients do not need to be admitted for a (regularly recurring) depressive episode but can be treated on an outpatient basis and can receive treatment and an intervention aimed at relapse prevention at home, with possibly better long-term effects. Or, for example, patients who receive specific wound care at home and do not need to visit a dermatologist because the nurse has regular contact with the dermatologist through telecare.

A basic idea in value-based healthcare is that if the quality of care is improved by the changes that have been initiated in healthcare, the efficiency will also increase. One example is the combination of advanced diagnostics, decision support systems, and shared decision-making.

Nursing patient-oriented leadership is necessary to continue to look at care with a patient-friendly view when the input for care processes is changed. An important advantage is that evidence-based healthcare provides nurses with feedback on their nursing actions. Which care is effective, which input to care leads to which effect, which input leads to which output to care? This feedback on nursing care can improve the effectiveness and the quality of care. This is not only in terms of cost-effectiveness—which is certainly important in an era of more and more people with chronic health problems—but also in terms of high-quality nursing care.

29.5   Conclusion

- Value-based healthcare is about outcomes, patient outcomes of care and treatment, and improving the patient's experienced quality of life.
- Value-based healthcare requires a multidisciplinary approach to care and treatment, with a focus on recovery rather than treatment per se.
- It also aims to limit healthcare costs by avoiding unnecessary procedures, shortening treatments and care, and making care and treatment less invasive for the patient.
- Nursing patient-oriented leadership is necessary to implement and maintain value-based healthcare, as it provides nurses with feedback on their nursing actions and improves the effectiveness and quality of care.
- Overall, a value-based orientation in healthcare is crucial for achieving better patient outcomes and improving the quality of care.

Box 29.1 Mind-Map Benefits of Value-Based Healthcare
Create a mind-map on the topic of "Value-Based Healthcare for Nursing Professionals."
   Point out what benefits patients may experience.
   Point out what the benefits are for nursing professionals.
   Put arrows between similarities.

Box 29.2 Mind-Map Value-Based Healthcare for Nursing Professionals
Create a mind-map on the topic of "Value-Based Healthcare for Nursing Professionals."

Objective: To understand the concept of value-based healthcare for nursing professionals and its importance in improving patient outcomes and reducing healthcare costs.

Instructions:

1. Write "Value-Based Healthcare for Nursing Professionals" in the center of the mind-map.
2. Add three branches to the center circle: "Definition," "Principles," and "Benefits."
3. Under the "Definition" branch, add sub-branches that explain what value-based healthcare is and how it differs from traditional healthcare.
4. Under the "Principles" branch, add sub-branches that outline the important principles associated with a value-based orientation on care, including patient-centered care, multidisciplinary approach, and focus on recovery.
5. Under the "Benefits" branch, add sub-branches that explain the benefits of value-based healthcare for patients, healthcare professionals, and healthcare organizations.
6. Add sub-branches under each principle and benefit to provide examples and further explanation.
7. Use colors, images, and symbols to make the mind-map more visually appealing and easier to understand.

References

Abdei-Tawab N, Roter D. The relevance of client-centered communication to family planning settings in developing countries: lessons from the Egyptian experience. Soc Sci Med. 2002;54:1357–68.

Abramson. 1985.

Arnold EC, Underman Boggs K. Interpersonal relationships. Professional communication skills for nurses. 8th ed. Amsterdam: Elsevier; 2020.

Atlantis E, Fahey P, Foster J. Collaborative care for comorbid depression and diabetes: a systematic review and meta-analysis. Patient-centred medicine. BMJ. 2014;4(4):e004706.

Baart A. De ontdekking van kwaliteit. SWP uitgeverij; 2018. ISBN: 9789088508349.

Barlem ELD, Ramos FRS. Constructing a theoretical model of moral distress. Nurs Ethics. 2014;22:608. https://doi.org/10.1177/0969733014551595.

Bass BM, Avolio BJ, Jung DI, Berson Y. Predicting unit performance by assessing transformational and transactional leadership. J Appl Psychol. 2003;88(2):207–18.

Bate P, Robert G. Experience-based design: from redesigning the system around the patient to co-designing services with the patient. Qual Saf Health Care. 2006;15:307–10. https://doi.org/10.1136/qshc.2005.016527. (This is based on mapping a consecutive series of 'touch points' between the patient and the service where patient experience is actively shaped).

Baum N. Moving from the Triple to the Quadruple Aim. The Journal of Medical Practice Management: MPM. 2021;36(6): 300–02.

Bergeson SC, Dean JD. A systems approach to patient-centered care. JAMA. 2006;296(23):2848–51. https://doi.org/10.1001/jama.296.23.2848.

Bertakis KD, Azari R. Patient-centered care is associated with decreased health care utilization. J Am Board Fam Med. 2011;24(3):229–39. https://doi.org/10.3122/jabfm.2011.03.100170.

Bodenheimer T, Sinsky C. From triple to quadruple aim: care of the patient requires care of the provider. Fam Med. 2014;12(6):573–6. https://doi.org/10.1370/afm.1713ann.

Boot JMD. Organisatie van de gezondheidszorg. Assen: Van Gorkum BV; 2018.

Boyle G. Autonomy in long-term care: a need, a right, or a luxury? Disabil Soc. 2008;23:299–310.

Bradshaw T, Pedley R. Evolving role of mental health nurses in the physical health care of people with serious mental health illness. Int J Ment Health Nurs. 2012;21(3):266–73. https://doi.org/10.1111/j.1447-0349.2012.00818.x.

Chen R, Atzil-Slonim C, et al. Therapists' recognition of alliance ruptures as a moderator of change in alliance and symptoms. Psychother Res. 2018;28:560.

Chewning B, Bylund CL, Shah B, Arora NK, Gueguen JA, Makoul G. Patient preferences for shared decisions: a systematic review. Patient Educ Couns. 2012;86(1):9–18. https://doi.org/10.1016/j.pec.2011.02.004.

Clavelle JT, Porter-O'Grady T, Weston MJ, Verran JA. Evolution of structural empowerment: moving from shared to professional governance. J Nurs Adm. 2016;46(6):308–12. https://doi.org/10.1097/nna.0000000000000350.

Cleary M, Horsfall J, Deacon M, Jackson D. Leadership and mental health nursing. Issues Ment Health Nurs. 2011;32(10):632.

Cleary M, Horsfall J, O'Hara-Aarons M, Jackson D, Hunt GE. Mental health nurses' perceptions of good work in an acute setting. Int J Ment Health Nurs. 2012a;21(5):471–9.

Cleary M, Hunt GE, Horsfall J, Deacon M. Nurse-patient interaction in acute adult inpatient mental health units: a review and synthesis of qualitative studies. Issues Ment Health Nurs. 2012b;33(2):66–79. Published online: 25 Jan 2012. https://doi.org/10.3109/0161284 0.2011.622428.

Cleary M, Horsfall J, O'Hara-Aarons M. Mental health nurses' views of recovery within an acute setting. Int J Ment Health Nurs. 2012c;22(3):205–12.

Conn LG, Lingard L, Reeves S, Miller K, Russell A, Zwarenstein M. Communication channels in general internal medicine: a description of baseline patterns for improved interprofessional communication. Qual Health Res. 2009;19(7):943–53.

Constand MK, MacDermid JC, Bello-Haas VD, Law M. Scoping review of patient-centered care approaches in healthcare. BMC Health Serv Res. 2014;14:271. https://doi.org/10.1186/1472-6963-14-271.

Coyne I, O'Neill C, Murphy M, Costello T, O'Shea R. What does family-centered care mean to nurses and how do they think it could be enhanced in practice. J Adv Nurs. 2011;67(12):2561–73.

Crawford MJ, Rutter D, Manley C, Weaver T, Bhui K, Fulop N, et al. Systematic review of involving patients in the planning and development of health care. BMJ. 2002;325(7375):1263. https://doi.org/10.1136/bmj.325.7375.1263.

Cummings G, Lee H, Macgregor T, Davey M, Wong C, Paul L, et al. Factors contributing to nursing leadership: a systematic review. J Health Serv Res Policy. 2008;13(4):240–8.

Davis K, Schoenbaum SC, Audet AM. A 2020 vision of patient-centered primary care. J Gen Intern Med. 2005;20:953–7.

Dixon JF, Larison K, Zabari M. Skilled communication: making it real. AACN Adv Crit Care. 2006;17(4):376–82.

Doyle C, Lennox L, Bell D. A systematic review of evidence on the links between patient experience and clinical safety and effectiveness. BMJ Open. 2013;3(1):1–18.

Dwamena F, Holmes-Rovner M, Gaulden CM, et al. Interventions for providers to promote a patient-centred approach in clinical consultations. Cochrane Database Syst Rev. 2012;(12):CD003267.

Edward H, Wagner BT. Austin and Michael Von Korff organizing care for patients with chronic illness. Milbank Q. 1996;74(4):511–44.

Ekman I, Swedberg K, Taft C, Lindseth A, Norberg A, Brink E, et al. Person-centered care—ready for prime time. Eur J Cardiovasc Nurs. 2011;10:248–51.

Elliss-Brookes L, McPhail S, Ives A, Greenslade M, Shelton J, Hiom S, et al. Routes to diagnosis for cancer—determining the patient journey using multiple routine data sets. Br J Cancer. 2012;107:1220–6.

Epstein RM, Street RL Jr. The values and value of patient-centered care. Ann Fam Med. 2011;9(2):100–3.

Eubanks CF, Burckell LA, et al. Clinical consensus strategies to repair ruptures in the therapeutic alliance. J Psychother Integr. 2017;28:60–76.

Eubanks C, Safran JD, Muran JC. Alliance rupture repair: a meta analysis. Psychotherapy. 2018;55:508–19.

Ferrell BR, Kravitz K, Borneman T, Friedmann ET. Family caregivers: a qualitative study to better understand the quality-of-life concerns and needs of this population. Clin J Oncol Nurs. 2018;22(3):286–94. 9p. 8 Charts.

Fischer SA. Transformational leadership in nursing: a concept analysis. J Adv Nurs. 2016;72:2644. https://doi.org/10.1111/jan.13049.

Fisher CH, Jabara J, Poudriers L, Williams T, Wallen G. Shared governance: the way to staff satisfaction and retention. Nurs Manag. 2016;47(11):14–6.

Fleming DA, et al. Caregiving at the end of life: perceptions of health care quality and quality of life among patients and caregivers. J Pain Symptom Manage. 2006;31(5):407–20.

Foronda C, MacWilliams B, McArthur E. Interprofessional communication in healthcare: an integrative review. Nurse Educ Pract. 2016;19:36–40.

Foronda CL, Walsh H, Budhathoki C. Evaluating nurse–physician communication with a rubric: a pilot study. J Contin Educ Nurs. 2019;50(4):163–9.

Freidson, Eliot. Professionalism, the third logic: On the practice of knowledge. University of Chicago press, 2001.

Gagliardi AR, Wright FC, Look Hong NJ, Groot G, Helyer L, Meiers P, et al. National consensus recommendations on patient-centered care for ductal carcinoma in situ. Breast Cancer Res Treat. 2019;174(3):561–70.

Gaydos HL. Understanding personal narratives: an approach to practice. J Adv Nurs. 2005;49:254.

Gerteis M, Edgman-Levitan S, Daley J, Delbanco TL. Through the patient's eyes. San Francisco: Jossey-Bass Publishers; 1993.

Gill SD, Gill M. Partnering with consumers: national standards and lessons from other countries. Med J Aust. 2015;203(3):134–6. https://doi.org/10.5694/mja14.01656.

Gill SD, Fuscaldo G, Page RS. Patient-centred care through a broader lens: supporting patient autonomy alongside moral deliberation. Emerg Med Australas. 2019;31(4):680–2. https://doi.org/10.1111/1742-6723.13287.

Giltinane CL. Leadership styles and theories. Nurs Stand. 2013;27(41):35–9.

Glasgow RE, Orleans CT, Wagner EH, Curry SJ, Solberg LI. Does the chronic care model serve also as a template for improving prevention? Milbank Q. 2003;79(4):579–612. First published: 06 June 2003. https://doi.org/10.1111/1468-0009.00222.

Goodwin N. Understanding integrated care: a complex process, a fundamental principle. Int J Integr Care. 2013;13:e011. URN:NBN:NL:UI:10-1-114416 1 Editorial.

Gray MF, Murray L, Abraham M, Nickel W, Sweeney JM, Frosch DL, et al. Actions and processes that patients, family members, and physicians associate with patient- and family-centered care. BMC Fam Pract. 2019;20:35. https://doi.org/10.1186/s12875-019-0918-7.

Gregory M. A possible patient journey: a tool to facilitate patient-centered care. New York, NY: Thieme Medical Publishers; 2012.

Haggerty J, Roberge D, Freeman G, Beaulieu C. Experienced continuity of care when patients see multiple clinicians: a qualitative metasummary. Ann Fam Med. 2013;11:262–71.

Happel B, Scott D. Should we or should we not? Mental health nurses' view on physical health care of mental health consumers. Ment Health Nurs. 2012;5(1):4–12.

Happell B, Scott D, Platania-Phung C, Nankivell J. Should we or shouldn't we? Mental health nurses' views on physical health care of mental health consumers. Int J Ment Health Nurs. 2012;21(3):202–10. https://doi.org/10.1111/j.1447-0349.2011.00799.x.

Heinen MM, Van Achterberg T, Schwendimann R, Zander B, Matthews A, Kózka M, et al. Nurses' intention to leave their profession: a cross sectional observational study in 10 European countries. Int J Nurs Stud. 2013;50(2):174–84. https://doi.org/10.1016/j.ijnurstu.2012.09.019.

Hirsch ES, Adler G, Amspoker AB, Williams JR, Marsh L. Improving detection of psychiatric disturbances in Parkinson's disease: the role of informants. J Parkinsons Dis. 2013;3:55–60.

Hobbs JH. A dimensional analysis of patient-centered care. Nurs Res. 2009;58:52–62.

Holland. 1994.

Horowitz A, Silverstone BM, Reinhardt JP. A conceptual and empirical exploration of personal autonomy issues within family caregiving relationships. Gerontologist. 1991;31:23–31.

Horsfall D, Paton J, Carrington A. Experiencing recovery: findings from a qualitative study into mental illness, self and place. J Ment Health. 2018;27(4):307–13. Received 19 Dec 2016, Accepted 14 Sep 2017. Published online: 05 Oct 2017. https://doi.org/10.1080/09638237.2017.1385736.

Hsu C, Gray MF, Murray L, Abraham M, Nickel W. Actions and processes that patients, family members, and physicians associate with patient- and family-centered care. BMC Fam Pract. 2019;20:35.

Hubble MA, Duncan BL, Miller SD. Directing attention to what works. In: Hubble MA, Duncan BL, Miller SD, editors. The heart and soul of change: what works in therapy. American Psychological Association; 1999. 407–47. https://doi.org/10.1037/11132-013.

Huber M, Staps S. Self-management for health and environment: time for a new approach-position paper. Louis Bolk Instituut en Institute for Positive Health White; 2016.

ICF, Nederlandse vertaling – WHO-ICF Collaborating Centre. IFC, Nederlandse vertaling van de 'international classification of functioning. disability and health'. Houten: Bohn Stafleu van Loghum; 2002.

Institute of Medicine. Crossing the quality chasm: a new health system for the 21st century. Washington, DC: National Academies Press; 2001.

Johnston R, Kong X. The customer experience: a road-map for improvement. Manag Serv Qual. 2011;21:5–24. https://doi.org/10.1108/09604521111100225.

Kenyon G. Narrative gerontology. New York: Wiley; 2015. https://doi.org/10.1002/9781118521373.wbeaa034.

Kitson A, Marshall A, Bassett K, Zeitz K. What are the core elements of patient-centred care? A narrative review and synthesis of the literature from health policy, medicine and nursing. J Adv Nurs. 2013;69(1):4–15.

Kogan AC, Wilber K, Mosqueda L. Person-centered care for older adults with chronic conditions and functional impairment: a systematic literature review. J Am Geriatr Soc. 2015;64:e1. https://doi.org/10.1111/jgs.13873.

Korhonen A, Kangasniemi M. 2013.

Kouzes JM, Posner BZ. The leadership challenge. Chichester: Jossey-Bass; 2008.

Kuipers SJ, Cramm JM, Nieboer AP. The importance of patient-centered care and co-creation of care for satisfaction with care and physical and social well-being of patients with multi-morbidity in the primary care setting. BMC Health Serv Res. 2019;19:13.

Kutney-Lee A, Germack H, Hatfield L. Nurse engagement in shared governance and patient and nurse outcomes. J Nurs Adm. 2016;46(11):605–12.

Laschinger H, Hall L, Pedersen C, Almost J. A psychometric analysis of the patient satisfaction with nursing care quality questionnaire: an actionable approach to measuring patient satisfaction. Nurs Care Qual. 2005;20:220–30.

Lawford BJ, Bennell KL, Kasza J, Campbell PK, Gale J, Bills C, Hinman RS. Implementation of person-centred practice principles and behaviour change techniques after a 2-day training workshop: a nested case study involving physiotherapists. Muscoskelet Care. 2019;17:221. https://doi.org/10.1002/msc.1395.

Lawrence D, Kisely S. Inequalities in healthcare provision for people with severe mental illness. J Psychopharmacol. 2010;24(4 Suppl):61–8.

Leplege A, et al. Person-centredness: conceptual and historical perspectives. Disabil Rehabil. 2007;29(20–21):1555–65.

Levinson W, Lesser CS, Epstein RM. Developing physician communication skills for patient-centered care. Health Aff. 2010;29(7):1310.

Liaw SY, Zhou WT, Lau TC, Siau C, Chan SW. An interprofessional communication training using simulation to enhance safe care for a deteriorating patient. Nurse Educ Today. 2014;34(2):259–64.

Lor M, Crooks N, Tluczek A. A proposed model of person-, family-, and culture-centered nursing care. Nurs Outlook. 2016;64(4):352–66.

Maizes V, Rakel D, Niemiec C. Integrative medicine and patient-centered care. Explore. 2009;5(5):277–89. https://doi.org/10.1016/j.explore.2009.06.008.

McCarthy S, O'Raghallaigh P, Woodworth S, Lin Lim Y, Kenny LC, Adam F. An integrated patient journey mapping tool for embedding quality in healthcare service reform. J Decis Syst. 2016;25:354–68. Published online: 16 Jun 2016. https://doi.org/10.1080/12460125.2016.1187394.

McCormack B. A conceptual framework for person-centred practice with older people. Int J Nurs Pract. 2003;9:202–9.

McCormack B, McCance T. Development of a framework for person-centred nursing. J Adv Nurs. 2006;56(5):1–8.

McCormack B, Karlsson B, Dewing J, Lerdal A. Exploring person-centredness: a qualitative meta-synthesis of four studies. Scand J Caring Sci. 2010;24(3):620–34. https://doi.org/10.1111/j.1471-6712.2010.00814.x.

McCormack LA, Treiman K, Rupert D, Williams-Piehota P, Nadler E, Arora NK, et al. Measuring patient-centered communication in cancer care: a literature review and the development of a systematic approach. Soc Sci Med. 2011;72:1085–95.

McEvoy L, Duffy A. Holistic practice—a concept analysis. Nurse Educ Pract. 2008;8(6):412–19.

Mead N, Bower P. Patient-centredness: a conceptual framework and review of the empirical literature. Soc Sci Med. 2000;51(7):1087–110.

Mill JS. Three essays. Oxford: Oxford University Press; 1975.

Molewijk B, Verkerk M, Milius H, Widdershoven G. Implementing moral case deliberation in a psychiatric hospital: process and outcome. Med Health Care Philos. 2008;11(1):43–56.

Morgan S, Yoder LH. A concept analysis of person-centered care. J Holist Nurs. 2012;30(1):6–15. https://doi.org/10.1177/0898010111412189.

Naef R, Ernst J, Petry H. Adaption, benefit and quality of care associated with primary nursing in an acute inpatient setting: a cross-sectional descriptive study. J Adv Nurs. 2019;75(10):2133–43. https://doi.org/10.1111/jan.13995. Epub 2019 Apr.

Naidu A. Factors affecting patient satisfaction and healthcare quality. Int J Health Care Qual Assur. 2009;22(4):366.

Oliveira VC, Refshauge KM, Ferreira ML, Pinto RZ, et al. Communication that values patient autonomy is associated with satisfaction with care: a systematic review. J Physiother. 2012;58(4):215–29.

Penny H and Jennifer G. Describing Nurse Leaders' and Direct Care Nurses' Perceptions of a Healthy Work Environment in Acute Care Settings, Part 2. The Journal of Nursing Administration. 2016;46(9):462–67. Published By: Lippincott Williams & Wilkins.

Peplau HE. Peplau's theory of interpersonal relations. Nurs Sci Q. 1997;10(4):162–7.

Perry AG, Potter PA, Ostendorf WR. Nursing interventions and clinical skills. 7th ed. Amsterdam: Elsevier; 2020.

Pickles J, Hide E, Maher L. Experience based design: a practical method of working with patients to redesign services. Clin Govern Int J. 2008;13:51–8.

Porter ME, Pabo EA, Lee TH. Redesigning primary care: a strategic vision to improve value by organizing around patients' needs. Health Aff. 2013;32(3):516.

Porter-O'Grady T. Researching shared governance. J Nurs Adm. 2003;33:251–2.

Ramon, et al. 2007.

Rastgardani T, Marras C, Gagliardi AR. Improving patient-centred care for persons with Parkinson's: qualitative interviews with care partners about their engagement in discussions of "off" periods. Health Expect. 2019;22:555. https://doi.org/10.1111/hex.12884.

Ratelle JT, Sawatsky AP, Kashiwagi DT, Schouten WM, Erwin PJ, Gonzalo JD, et al. Implementing bedside rounds to improve patient-centred outcomes: a systematic review. BMJ Qual Saf. 2017;28(4):317–26. https://doi.org/10.1136/bmjqs-2017-007778.

Rathert C, Wyrwich MD, Boren SA. Patient-centered care and outcomes: a systematic review of the literature. Med Care Res Rev. 2013;70(4):351. https://doi.org/10.1177/1077558712465774.

Rogers CR. On becoming a person. New York, NY: Houghton Mifflin; 1961.

Rosland AM, Heisler M, Piette JD. The impact of family behaviors and communication patterns on chronic illness outcomes: a systematic review. J Behav Med. 2012;35(2):221–39.

Safran DG, Miller W, Beckman H. Organizational dimensions of relationship-centered care theory, evidence, and practice. J Gen Intern Med. 2006;21(Suppl 1):S9–S15. https://doi.org/10.1111/j.1525-1497.2006.00303.x. PMCID: PMC1484831; PMID: 16405711.

Sassen B. Gezondheidsbevordering en zelfmanagement door verpleegkundigen en verpleegkundig specialisten. Houten: Bohn Stafleu van Loghum; 2018a. p. 9789036820110.

Sassen B. Nursing: health education and improving patient self-management. Berlin: Springer; 2018b. ISBN: 9783319517681.

Sassen B. Nursing: Health education and improving patient self-management. Intervention Mapping for healthy lifestyles. Berlin: Springer; 2023. ISBN: 9783031112546.

Scholl I, Zill JM, Harter M, Dirmaier J. An integrative model of patient-centeredness—a systematic review and concept analysis. PLoS One. 2014;9(9):e107828.

Sitvast J. Recovery in mental health care with the aid of photo-stories: an action research based on the principles of hermeneutic photography. Nurs Health. 2015;3(6):139–46.

Stewart M, Brown JB, Donner A, McWhinney IR, Oates J, Weston WW, et al. The impact of patient-centered care on outcomes. Fam Pract. 2000;49(9):796–804.

Suhonen R, Välimäki M, Katajisto J. Developing and testing an instrument for the measurement of individual care. J Adv Nurs. 2000;32:1253–63.

Suhonen R, Välimäki M, Leino-Kilpi H. Individualised care from patients', nurses' and relatives' perspective—a review of the literature. Int J Nurs Stud. 2002;39:645–54.

Sulmasy DP. A biopsychosocial-spiritual model for the care of patients at the end of life. Gerontologist. 2002;42(Suppl 3):24–33. https://doi.org/10.1093/geront/42.suppl_3.24.

Thompson J. Transformational leadership can improve workforce competencies. Nurs Manag. 2012;18(10):21–4.

Thompson L, McCabe R. The effect of clinician-patient alliance and communication on treatment adherence in mental health care: a systematic review. BMC Psychiatry. 2012;12:87.

Thota AB, Sipe TA, Byard GJ, Zometa CS, Hahn RA, McKnight-Eily LR, et al. Community preventive services task force collaborative care to improve the management of depressive disorders: a community guide systematic review and meta-analysis. Am J Prev Med. 2012;42(5):525–38.

Tornøe KA, Danbolt LJ, Kvigne K, Sørlie V. The power of consoling presence—Hospice nurses' lived experience with spiritual and existential care for the dying. BMC Nurs. 2014;13:25. https://doi.org/10.1186/1472-6955-13-25.

Trebble TM, Hansi N, Hydes T, Smith MA, Baker M. Process mapping the patient journey: an introduction. BMJ. 2010;341:c4078. https://doi.org/10.1136/bmj.c4078.

Tregunno D, Jeffs L, McGillis Hall L, Baker R, Doran D, Bassett S. On the ball—leadership for patient safety and learning in critical care. J Nurs Adm. 2009;39(7/8):334–9.

Tuominen L, Meretoja R, Leino-Kilpi H, Stolt M, Meretoja R, Leino-Kilpi H. Effectiveness of nursing interventions among patients with cancer: an overview of systematic reviews. J Clin Nurs. 2018;28(13–14):2401–19. https://doi.org/10.1111/jocn.14762.

Urden LD, Stacy KM, Lough ME. Priorities in critical care nursing. 8th ed. Amsterdam: Elsevier; 2020.

Vaismoradi M, Kangasniemi SJM. Patient participation in patient safety and nursing input—a systematic review. J Clin Nurs. 2014;24:627. https://doi.org/10.1111/jocn.12664.

Valentijn PP, Schepman SM, Opheij W, Bruijnzeels MA. Understanding integrated care: a comprehensive conceptual framework based on the integrative functions of primary care. Int J Integr Care. 2013;22(13):e010.

Van Achterberg T, Schoonhoven L, Grol R. Nursing implementation science: how evidence-based nursing requires evidence-based implementation. J Nurs Scholarsh. 2008;40(4):302–10. https://doi.org/10.1111/j.1547-5069.2008.00243.x.

Van Straten A, Hill J, Richards DA, Cuijpers P. Stepped care treatment delivery for depression: a systematic review and meta-analysis. Psychol Med. 2014;45:231. https://doi.org/10.1017/S0033291714000701.

Ventegodt S, Kandel I, Ervin DA, Merrick J. Health care for people with intellectual and developmental disabilities across the lifespan. Cham: Springer; 2016. p. 1935–41.

Vermoch KL, Bunting RF. Benchmarking patient- and family-centered care: highlights from a study of practices in 26 academic medical centers. Patient Saf. 2010;30:4. https://doi.org/10.1002/jhrm.20047.

Vlek H, Driessen S, Hassink L. Confronting the quality paradox: towards new characterisations of 'quality' in contemporary healthcare. BMC Health Serv Res. 2013;15:240–6.

Wagner EH, Austin BT, Von Korff M. Organizing care for patients with chronic illness. Milbank Q. 1996;74(4):511–44.

Watzlawick p, Weakland JH, Fisch R. Principles of problem formation and problem resolution. 2011.

Weidema FC, Molewijk AC, Widdershoven GAM, Abma TA. Enacting ethics: bottom-up involvement in implementing moral case deliberation. Health Care Anal. 2012;20(1):1–19.

Weiss T, Swede MJ. Transforming preprofessional health education through relationship-centered care and narrative medicine. Teach Learn Med. 2019;31(2):222–33. Published online: 04 May 2016. https://doi.org/10.1080/10401334.2016.1159566.

Welford C, Murphy K, Rodgers V, Frauenlob T. Autonomy for older people in residential care: a selective literature review. Int J Older People Nurs. 2012;7(1):65–9.

Wessel S, Abelson D, Manthey M. Care delivery design that holds patients and families. In: Advancing relationship-based cultures. Minneapolis (MN): Creative Health Care Management; 2017. p. 201–21.

WHO. Adherence to long-term therapies. Evidence for action. Geneva: WHO; 2003. ISBN 9241545992.

Wong CA, Cummings GG, Ducharme L. The relationship between nursing leadership and patient outcomes: a systematic review update. J Nurs Manag. 2013;21:709–24.

Yamanishi T, Tachibana H, Oguru M, et al. Anxiety and depression in patients with Parkinson's disease. Intern Med. 2013;52(5):539–45.

Ying AI, Feeley TW, Porter ME. Value-based healthcare: implications for thyroid cancer. Health Aff. 2016; 32(3). Promoting Health & Wellness Published Online: 8 Apr 2016. https://doi.org/10.2217/ije-2015-0005.

Yoder-Wisse PS. Leading and managing in nursing. 7th ed tion. Elsevier, 2019. isbn 9780323449137

Yun DW, Choi JS. Person-centered rehabilitation care and outcomes: a systematic literature review. Int J Nurs Stud. 2019;93:74–83. https://www.sciencedirect.com/science/article/pii/S0020748919300537?casa_token=Rza59F4UlyIAAAAA:-AS5Nl%2D%2DcqcUU1yCJvXAR9SZCaW86L0bs7bJZzEWLKkrpNiM6Fw143fFIzLM9RMhdWqPPzmz_HQ.

Yusof MM, Kuljis J, Papazafeiropoulou A, Stergioulas LK. An evaluation framework for health information systems: human, organization and technology-fit factors (HOT-fit). Int J Med Inform. 2008;77:386–98. https://doi.org/10.1016/j.ijmedinf.2007.08.011.

Zamanzadeh V, Jasemi M, Valizadeh L, Keogh B, Taleghani F. Effective factors in providing holistic care: a qualitative study. Indian J Pallat Care. 2015;21(2):214–24. https://doi.org/10.4103/0973-1075.156506. PMCID: PMC4441185; PMID: 26009677.

Further Reading

Aiken LH, Sloane DM, Bruyneel L, Van den Heede K, Griffiths P, Busse R, et al. Nurse staffing and education and hospital mortality in nine European countries: a retrospective observational study. Lancet. 2014;383(9931):1824–30. https://doi.org/10.1016/S0140-6736(13)62631-8.

Boyles CM, Bailey PH, Mossey S. Representations of disability in nursing and healthcare literature: an integrative review. J Adv Nurs. 2008;62(4):428–37.

Celentano DD, Szklo M. Gordis epidemiology. 6th ed. Amsterdam: Elsevier; 2019a.

Celentano DD, Szklo M. Gordis. Epidemiología. Elsevier; 2019b.

Clark PG. Narrative in interprofessional education and practice: implications for professional identity, provider–patient communication and teamwork. J Interprof Care. 2014a;28(1):34–9.

Clark R. Cognitive task analysis for expert-based instruction in healthcare. In: Handbook of research on educational communications and technology; 2014b. p. 541–51.

Coyne I, Harder M. Children's participation in decision-making: balancing protection with shared decision-making using a situational perspective. J Child Health Care. 2011;15(4):312–9.

Dixon A, Le Grand J. Is greater patient choice consistent with equity? The case of the English NHS. J Health Serv Res Policy. 2006;11(3):162–6.

Gill SD, Lane SE, Sheridan M, Ellis E, Smith D, Stella J. Why do 'fast track' patients stay more than four hours in the emergency department? An investigation of factors that predict length of stay. Emerg Med Australas. 2018;30:641. https://doi org/10.1111/1742-6723.12964.

Grant M, Opie J, Friedman D, Hughes A. Inpatient electronic handover notes as a relevant interim discharge information package for general practitioners. Aust J Gen Pract. 2015;44(10):698.

Kenning C, Fisher L, Bee P, Bower P, Coventry P. Primary care practitioner and patient understanding of the concepts of multimorbidity and self-management: a qualitative study. SAGE Open Med. 2013;1:2050312113510001.

Lipkin M Jr, Quill TE, Napodano RJ. The medical interview: a core curriculum for residencies in internal medicine. Ann Intern Med. 1984;100(2):277–84.

Oandasan IF, Conn LG, Lingard L, Karim A, Jakubovicz D, Whitehead C, et al. The impact of space and time on interprofessional teamwork in Canadian primary health care settings: implications for health care reform. Prim Health Care Res Dev. 2009;10(2):151–62.

Roberts JP, Fisher TR, Trowbridge MJ, Bent C. A design thinking framework for healthcare management and innovation. Healthcare. 2016;4(1):11–4. Elsevier.

Index

Printed in the United States
by Baker & Taylor Publisher Services